THE PLANT-BASED DIET FOR SINGLE

2 Books in 1: Live a Healthy Lifestyle and Lose Rapidly Weight with a Large Choice of 240+ Vegan and Vegetarian Recipes! Special Guide Included!

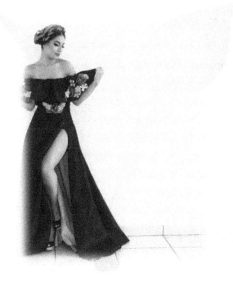

By

Audrey Pottery

TABLE OF CONTENT

PART 1-INTRODUCTION: THE BENEFITS PLANT-BASED DIET

A plant-based diet has proven health effects due to its food composition. Reduced saturated fat consumption prevents various diseases, including cardiovascular problems, high cholesterol levels, and obesity. The following are other guaranteed benefits of this diet:

WEIGHT AND BMI CONTROL

Research studies conducted on the plant-based diet have revealed that people who follow it tend to have a lower BMI or body mass index, reduced risk of obesity, and a lower likelihood of heart disease and diabetes. This is mainly because plant-based diets provide more fiber, water, and carbohydrates to the body. This can keep the body's metabolism active and functioning properly while providing a good boost of continuous energy.

In 2018, a study was conducted on this diet plan, and it was found to be the most effective in treating obesity. In that study, 75 people with obesity or weight issues were given a completely vegan plant-based diet, and their results were compared to those consuming animal-based diets. After four months of this experiment, the plant-based diet group showed a significant decrease in their body weight (up to 6.5 kilograms). Everyone lost more fat mass and demonstrated improved insulin sensitivity. Another study involving 60,000 individuals showed similar results, with people following a vegan diet recording lower body mass index than vegetarians and those following a plant-based diet.

Lower risk of heart disease and other conditions

The American Heart Association recently conducted a study in which middle-aged adults who followed a plant-based diet were studied. All of the subjects showed a decrease in their rate of heart disease. Based on the results of this research, the association listed the following illnesses that can be prevented through a plant-based diet:

- Heart attack
- Certain types of cancer
- Diabetes
- High blood pressure
- Type II diabetes
- High cholesterol levels
- Obesity

Plant-based diets also help manage diabetes because they improve insulin sensitivity and combat insulin resistance. Of all 60,000 study participants, about 2.9% on the vegan diet had type II diabetes, while 7.6% of participants on non-vegetarian diets had type II diabetes. From this observation, the researchers confirmed that a plant-based diet could help in the treatment of diabetes. It has also been proposed that this diet may help diabetic patients lose weight, improve metabolic rate and decrease their need for medical treatment.

It has also been suggested that doctors recommend this diet as part of treating people with type II diabetes or prediabetes. While medical treatments ensure short-term results, the plant-based dietary approach offers long-term results.

WHAT CAN I EAT?

There is a long list of foods allowed on the plant-based diet, including grains, fruits, vegetables, legumes, seeds, oils, and nuts. Here are detailed lists of some of the foods that you can freely consume in the plant-based diet.

FRUITS

Since all fruits come from plants, they are all safe to eat while on a plant-based diet. This is different from other popular diets that do not allow most fruits due to their sugar content. Some fruits that can be enjoyed are:

- Apples
- Citrus fruits
- Berries

- Bananas
- Grapes
- Melons

- avocados

VEGETABLES

Other diets are restrictive on the types of vegetables allowed; the plant-based diet includes all vegetables without any restrictions. However, fiber-rich vegetables are preferred, especially green leafy vegetables that are rich in minerals and vitamins. Some vegetables that you can safely eat on a plant-based diet are:

- Cauliflower
- Broccoli
- Kale

- Beet
- Asparagus
- Carrot

- tomatoes
- Peppers
- Zucchinis

Other vegetables are rich in carbohydrates and vitamins. These are also allowed in this diet. They include most root vegetables, including:

- Potatoes
- Beets

- Sweet Potato
- Butternut squash

LEGUMES

Legumes are a vital and fundamental part of the plant-based diet. They greatly compliment other plant-based ingredients as they are rich in both carbohydrates, protein, and vitamins. Legumes are the underground part of a plant used to store most of its nutrients, which is why they are so beneficial. Examples of these are:

- Black beans
- Chickpeas

- Lentils
- Peas

- Kidney Beans

SEEDS

Seeds, even if consumed in a tiny amount, provide many vitamins and minerals. For example, sesame seeds contain a significant amount of vitamin E. Other seeds allowed in the plant-based diet are:

- Pumpkin seeds
- Chia seeds

- Hemp seeds
- Flax seeds

WALNUTS

Like seeds, nuts are an essential source of all vitamins, healthy fats, and antioxidants. Here's a list of nuts allowed in the plant-based diet:

- Almonds
- Brazil nuts
- Macadamia nuts
- Pecans
- Cashews
- Pistachios

HEALTHY FATS

The best part of the plant-based diet is the healthy unsaturated fats allowed. They protect the body from bad cholesterol and resulting heart disease. Plant-based oils are permitted:

- Avocado oil
- Hemp seed oil
- Canola oil
- Walnut oil
- Flaxseed oil
- Chia seed oil
- Olive oil

WHOLE GRAINS

Another source of carbohydrates, whole grains, is also rich in minerals and fiber. They can help maintain blood sugar levels and are a vital part of this healthy diet. Here are all the whole grains used in this diet:

- Brown rice
- Buckwheat
- Rye
- Oats
- Quinoa
- Barley
- Spelt
- Whole wheat bread

Products made from or extracted from these whole grains can also be used in this diet, including flours, full-grain meals, etc.

VEGETABLE MILK

Since animal milk is not allowed in the plant-based diet, there are other plant-based options you can eat, including:

- Soy milk
- Coconut milk
- Almond Milk
- Rice milk
- Oat milk
- Almond milk
- Hemp milk

All of these kinds of milk have their distinct taste and texture and should be used accordingly. Look for unsweetened varieties for universal use.

FOOD TO AVOID

It has been established that all animal foods are not allowed in the plant-based diet, but other products are not allowed in a plant-based diet. Here is a detailed list:
- Animal meat: poultry, seafood, pork, lamb, and beef
- Butter, ghee, and other solid animal fats
- All processed foods
- Sugary foods such as cookies, cakes, and pastries
- All refined white carbohydrates
- Processed vegan and vegetarian alternatives that may contain added salt or sugar
- Excessive salt
- Fried foods

EIGHT FOOD-BASED MISTAKES

Without a clear understanding of the diet, people can make some mistakes while following a plant-based diet. This is mainly due to the subtle differences between the ingredients. The following are common food mistakes that people usually make and the different ways to avoid them:

BREAD

There are countless varieties of bread available today. While all loaves are made primarily from a basic flour batter, many additional ingredients can compromise the plant-based diet. The addition of butter, animal milk, fat or other animal products, or an excess of sugar and salt can make bread unsuitable for a plant-based diet. Be sure to double-check the ingredients in store-bought bread or make your bread at home using only vegan ingredients.

BROTH FOR SOUPS

Broths are commonly used in soups and curries, but most are liquid extracts of bones, meat, and vegetables. Because chicken and beef broths are usually used in popular soup recipes, people also use them in a plant-based diet. Vegetable broths and stocks should be used instead. The broth gets most of its nutrients and fat from the meat or bones in which it is cooked, so only vegetable broths are recommended for this diet.

PASTA

Whole wheat or basic flour pasta is an excellent option for enjoying some flavor and variety in your plant-based diet. Adding pasta to your plant-based menu is not harmful, but if the same pasta is cooked with animal ingredients, it is not suitable for this diet. Plant-based pasta recipes, including zucchini spaghetti, are also an excellent option for this diet.

ORANGE JUICE

Freshly squeezed organic orange juice is not nasty for the plant-based diet. It is a good source of vitamin C. However, when the juice is processed to add additional nutrients, the problem begins. Some companies add vitamin D2 or D3 to the juice. While vitamin D2 comes from plants, vitamin D3 is an animal-based vitamin not allowed in a plant-based diet. Read labels and do your research to avoid such products. It's best to rely on homemade, freshly squeezed juices rather than store-bought ones.

GRANOLA

Granola comes in a wide variety. Because of the diversity of ingredients used in different granola recipes, a person on a plant-based diet should be more careful in their selection. Granola may contain dairy products such as milk, butter, or eggs. These should be avoided completely. Instead, choose one made from oats, nuts, seeds, and vegetable fats while following this diet.

CREAMS AND CUSTARDS

Since all creams and cream cheeses are made from animal milk, they are prohibited in a plant-based diet, even in small amounts. Instead, non-dairy, plant-based creams should be used. Ointments made from soy or coconut milk taste good and have a rich, thick texture, just like other creams.

CHEESE

Cheese is a staple in most diets, but they are animal-based and now allowed, as mentioned above. This is where vegan cheeses come in. These cheeses are made with plant-based ingredients, including soy, nuts, tapioca, coconut, root vegetables, or aquafaba. Like dairy cheese, vegan cheese varies in shape, texture, and taste but provides a good substitute for animal-based cheese.

VEGAN SAUSAGES AND BURGERS

Burgers and sausages are commonly enjoyed and hard to pass up. Fortunately, now both burgers and sausages are available in plant-based varieties. These burgers and sausages look more like meat-based burgers and sausages but are made of shredded vegetables and batter. Always opt for these varieties while following a plant-based diet.

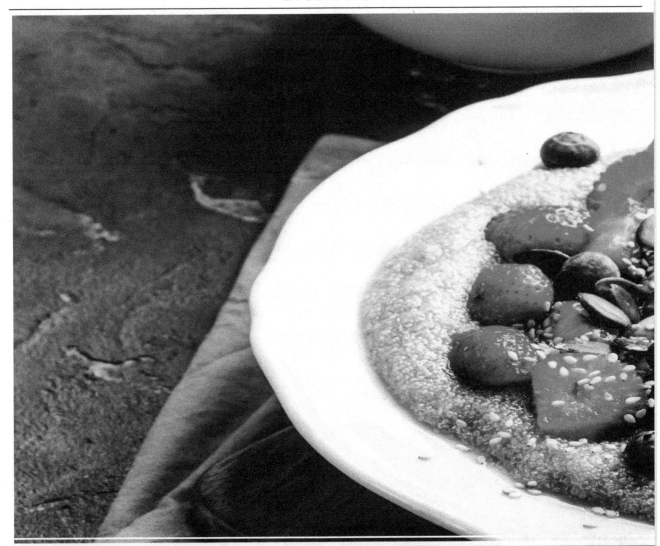

BREAKFAST

1) ORANGE CREPES

Preparation Time: 30 minutes   **Servings: 4**

Ingredients:

- ✓ 2 tbsp flax seed powder
- ✓ 1 tsp vanilla extract
- ✓ 1 tsp pure date sugar
- ✓ ¼ tsp salt
- ✓ 2 cups almond flour
- ✓ 1 ½ cups oat milk
- ✓ ½ cup melted plant butter
- ✓ 3 tbsp fresh orange juice
- ✓ 3 tbsp plant butter for frying

Directions:

- ❖ In a medium bowl, mix the flax seed powder with 6 tbsp water and allow thickening for 5 minutes to make the vegan "flax egg." Whisk in the vanilla, date sugar, and salt.
- ❖ Pour in a quarter cup of almond flour and whisk, then a quarter cup of oat milk, and mix until no lumps remain. Repeat the mixing process with the remaining almond flour and almond milk in the same quantities until exhausted.
- ❖ Mix in the plant butter, orange juice, and half of the water until the mixture is runny like pancakes. Add the remaining water until the mixture is lighter. Brush a non-stick skillet with some butter and place over medium heat to melt.
- ❖ Pour 1 tbsp of the batter into the pan and swirl the skillet quickly and all around to coat the pan with the batter. Cook until the batter is dry and golden brown beneath, about 30 seconds.
- ❖ Use a spatula to flip the crepe and cook the other side until golden brown too. Fold the crepe onto a plate and set aside. Repeat making more crepes with the remaining batter until exhausted. Drizzle some maple syrup on the crepes and serve

2) OAT BREAD WITH COCONUT

Preparation Time: 50 minutes   **Servings: 4**

Ingredients:

- ✓ 4 cups whole-wheat flour
- ✓ ¼ tsp salt
- ✓ ½ cup rolled oats
- ✓ 1 tsp baking soda
- ✓ 1 ¾ cups coconut milk, thick
- ✓ 2 tbsp pure maple syrup

Directions:

- ❖ Preheat the oven to 400 F.
- ❖ In a bowl, mix flour, salt, oats, and baking soda. Add in coconut milk and maple syrup and whisk until dough forms. Dust your hands with some flour and knead the dough into a ball. Shape the dough into a circle and place on a baking sheet.
- ❖ Cut a deep cross on the dough and bake in the oven for 15 minutes at 450 F. Reduce the temperature to 400 F and bake further for 20 to 25 minutes or until a hollow sound is made when the bottom of the bread is tapped. Slice and serve

3) ALMOND AND RAISIN GRANOLA

Preparation Time: 20 minutes   **Servings: 8**

Ingredients:

- ✓ 5 ½ cups old-fashioned oats
- ✓ 1 ½ cups chopped walnuts
- ✓ ½ cup shelled sunflower seeds
- ✓ 1 cup golden raisins
- ✓ 1 cup shaved almonds
- ✓ 1 cup pure maple syrup
- ✓ ½ tsp ground cinnamon
- ✓ ¼ tsp ground allspice
- ✓ A pinch of salt

Directions:

- ❖ Preheat oven to 325 F. In a baking dish, place the oats, walnuts, and sunflower seeds. Bake for 10 minutes.
- ❖ Lower the heat from the oven to 300 F. Stir in the raisins, almonds, maple syrup, cinnamon, allspice, and salt. Bake for an additional 15 minutes. Allow cooling before serving

4) PECAN AND PUMPKIN SEED OAT JARS

Preparation Time: 10 minutes + chilling time   **Servings: 5**

Ingredients:

- ✓ 2 ½ cups old-fashioned rolled oats
- ✓ 5 tbsp pumpkin seeds
- ✓ 5 tbsp chopped pecans
- ✓ 5 cups unsweetened soy milk
- ✓ 2 ½ tsp agave syrup
- ✓ Salt to taste
- ✓ 1 tsp ground cardamom
- ✓ 1 tsp ground ginger

Directions:

- ❖ • In a bowl, put oats, pumpkin seeds, pecans, soy milk, agave syrup, salt, cardamom, and ginger and toss to combine. Divide the mixture between mason jars. Seal the lids and transfer to the fridge to soak for 10-12 hours

5) EASY APPLE MUFFINS

Preparation Time: 40 minutes   **Servings: 4**

Ingredients:

- ✓ For the muffins:
- ✓ 1 flax seed powder + 3 tbsp water
- ✓ 1 ½ cups whole-wheat flour
- ✓ ¾ cup pure date sugar
- ✓ 2 tsp baking powder
- ✓ ¼ tsp salt
- ✓ 1 tsp cinnamon powder
- ✓ 1/3 cup melted plant butter
- ✓ 1/3 cup flax milk
- ✓ 2 apples, chopped
- ✓ For topping:
- ✓ 1/3 cup whole-wheat flour
- ✓ ½ cup pure date sugar
- ✓ ½ cup cold plant butter, cubed
- ✓ 1 ½ tsp cinnamon powder

Directions:

- ❖ Preheat oven to 400 F and grease 6 muffin cups with cooking spray. In a bowl, mix the flax seed powder with water and allow thickening for 5 minutes to make the vegan "flax egg."
- ❖ In a bowl, mix flour, date sugar, baking powder, salt, and cinnamon powder. Whisk in the butter, vegan "flax egg," flax milk, and fold in the apples. Fill the muffin cups two-thirds way up with the batter.
- ❖ In a bowl, mix remaining flour, date sugar, cold butter, and cinnamon powder. Sprinkle the mixture on the muffin batter. Bake for 20 minutes. Remove the muffins onto a wire rack, allow cooling, and serve

6) ALMOND YOGURT WITH BERRIES AND WALNUTS

Preparation Time: 10 minutes   **Servings: 4**

Ingredients:

- ✓ 4 cups almond milk
- ✓ Dairy-Free yogurt, cold
- ✓ 2 tbsp pure malt syrup
- ✓ 2 cups mixed berries, chopped
- ✓ ¼ cup chopped toasted walnuts

Directions:

- ❖ In a medium bowl, mix the yogurt and malt syrup until well-combined. Divide the mixture into 4 breakfast bowls. Top with the berries and walnuts. Enjoy immediately

7) BREAKFAST BLUEBERRY MUESLI

Preparation Time: 10 minutes   **Servings: 5**

Ingredients:

- ✓ 2 cups spelt flakes
- ✓ 2 cups puffed cereal
- ✓ ¼ cup sunflower seeds
- ✓ ¼ cup almonds
- ✓ ¼ cup raisins
- ✓ ¼ cup dried cranberries
- ✓ ¼ cup chopped dried figs
- ✓ ¼ cup shredded coconut
- ✓ ¼ cup non-dairy chocolate chips
- ✓ 3 tsp ground cinnamon
- ✓ ½ cup coconut milk
- ✓ ½ cup blueberries

Directions:

- ❖ • In a bowl, combine the spelt flakes, puffed cereal, sunflower seeds, almonds, raisins, cranberries, figs, coconut, chocolate chips, and cinnamon. Toss to mix well. Pour in the coconut milk. Let sit for 1 hour and serve topped with blueberries

8) BERRY AND ALMOND BUTTER SWIRL BOWL

Preparation Time: 10 minutes

Servings: 3

Ingredients:

- ✓ 1 ½ cups almond milk
- ✓ 2 small bananas
- ✓ 2 cups mixed berries, fresh or frozen
- ✓ 3 dates, pitted
- ✓ 3 scoops hemp protein powder
- ✓ 3 tbsp smooth almond butter
- ✓ 2 tbsp pepitas

Directions:

- ❖ In your blender or food processor, mix the almond milk with the bananas, berries and dates.
- ❖ Process until everything is well combined. Divide the smoothie between three bowls.
- ❖ Top each smoothie bowl with almond butter and use a butter knife to swirl the almond butter into the top of each smoothie bowl.
- ❖ Afterwards, garnish each smoothie bowl with pepitas, serve well-chilled and enjoy

9) OATS WITH COCONUT AND STRAWBERRIES

Preparation Time: 15 minutes

Servings: 2

Ingredients:

- ✓ 1/2 tbsp coconut oil
- ✓ 1 cup rolled oats
- ✓ A pinch of flaky sea salt
- ✓ 1/8 tsp grated nutmeg
- ✓ 1/4 tsp cardamom
- ✓ 1 tbsp coconut sugar
- ✓ 1 cup coconut milk, sweetened
- ✓ 1 cup water
- ✓ 2 tbsp coconut flakes
- ✓ 4 tbsp fresh strawberries

Directions:

- ❖ In a saucepan, melt the coconut oil over a moderate flame. Then, toast the oats for about 3 minutes, stirring continuously.
- ❖ Add in the salt, nutmeg, cardamom, coconut sugar, milk and water; continue to cook for 12 minutes more or until cooked through.
- ❖ Spoon the mixture into serving bowls; top with coconut flakes and fresh strawberries. Enjoy

10) BEST CHOCOLATE GRANOLA

Preparation Time: 1 hour

Servings: 10

Ingredients:

- ✓ 1/2 cup coconut oil
- ✓ 1/2 cup agave syrup
- ✓ 1 tsp vanilla paste
- ✓ 3 cups rolled oats
- ✓ 1/2 cup hazelnuts, chopped
- ✓ 1/2 cup pumpkin seeds
- ✓ 1/2 tsp ground cardamom
- ✓ 1 tsp ground cinnamon
- ✓ 1/4 tsp ground cloves
- ✓ 1 tsp Himalayan salt
- ✓ 1/2 cup dark chocolate, cut into chunks

Directions:

- ❖ Begin by preheating your oven to 260 degrees F; line two rimmed baking sheets with a piece parchment paper.
- ❖ Then, thoroughly combine the coconut oil, agave syrup and vanilla in a mixing bowl.
- ❖ Gradually add in the oats, hazelnuts, pumpkin seeds and spices; toss to coat well. Spread the mixture out onto the prepared baking sheets.
- ❖ Bake in the middle of the oven, stirring halfway through the cooking time, for about 1 hour or until golden brown.
- ❖ Stir in the dark chocolate and let your granola cool completely before storing. Store in an airtight container.
- ❖ Enjoy

11) PUMPKIN GRIDDLE CAKES AUTUMN SEASON

Preparation Time: 30 minutes

Servings: 4

Ingredients:

- ✓ 1/2 cup oat flour
- ✓ 1/2 cup whole-wheat white flour
- ✓ 1 tsp baking powder
- ✓ 1/4 tsp Himalayan salt
- ✓ 1 tsp sugar
- ✓ 1/2 tsp ground allspice
- ✓ 1/2 tsp ground cinnamon
- ✓ 1/2 tsp crystalized ginger
- ✓ 1 tsp lemon juice, freshly squeezed
- ✓ 1/2 cup almond milk
- ✓ 1/2 cup pumpkin puree
- ✓ 2 tbsp coconut oil

Directions:

- ❖ In a mixing bowl, thoroughly combine the flour, baking powder, salt, sugar and spices. Gradually add in the lemon juice, milk and pumpkin puree.
- ❖ Heat an electric griddle on medium and lightly slick it with the coconut oil.
- ❖ Cook your cake for approximately 3 minutes until the bubbles form; flip it and cook on the other side for 3 minutes longer until browned on the underside.
- ❖ Repeat with the remaining oil and batter. Serve dusted with cinnamon sugar, if desired. Enjoy

12) MUFFINS WITH TOFU ENGLISH RECIPE

Preparation Time: 15 minutes

Servings: 4

Ingredients:

- ✓ 2 tbsp olive oil
- ✓ 16 ounces extra-firm tofu
- ✓ 1 tbsp nutritional yeast
- ✓ 1/4 tsp turmeric powder
- ✓ 2 handfuls fresh kale, chopped
- ✓ Kosher salt and ground black pepper, to taste
- ✓ 4 English muffins, cut in half
- ✓ 4 tbsp ketchup
- ✓ 4 slices vegan cheese

Directions:

- ❖ Heat the olive oil in a frying skillet over medium heat. When it's hot, add the tofu and sauté for 8 minutes, stirring occasionally to promote even cooking.
- ❖ Add in the nutritional yeast, turmeric and kale and continue sautéing an additional 2 minutes or until the kale wilts. Season with salt and pepper to taste.
- ❖ Meanwhile, toast the English muffins until crisp.
- ❖ To assemble the sandwiches, spread the bottom halves of the English muffins with ketchup; top them with the tofu mixture and vegan cheese; place the bun topper on, close the sandwiches and serve warm.
- ❖ Enjoy

13) CINNAMON SEMOLINO PORRIDGE

Preparation Time: 20 minutes

Servings: 3

Ingredients:

- ✓ 3 cups almond milk
- ✓ 3 tbsp maple syrup
- ✓ 3 tsp coconut oil
- ✓ 1/4 tsp kosher salt
- ✓ 1/2 tsp ground cinnamon
- ✓ 1 ¼ cups semolina

Directions:

- ❖ In a saucepan, heat the almond milk, maple syrup, coconut oil, salt and cinnamon over a moderate flame.
- ❖ Once hot, gradually stir in the semolina flour. Turn the heat to a simmer and continue cooking until the porridge reaches your preferred consistency.
- ❖ Garnish with your favorite toppings and serve warm. Enjoy

14) APPLESAUCE DECADENT FRENCH TOAST

Preparation Time: 15 minutes

Servings: 1

Ingredients:

- ✓ 1/4 cup oat milk, sweetened
- ✓ 2 tbsp applesauce, sweetened
- ✓ 1/2 tsp vanilla paste
- ✓ A pinch of salt
- ✓ A pinch of grated nutmeg
- ✓ 1/4 tsp ground cloves
- ✓ 1/4 tsp ground cinnamon
- ✓ 2 slices rustic day-old bread slices
- ✓ 1 tbsp coconut oil
- ✓ 1 tbsp maple syrup

Directions:

- ❖ In a mixing bowl, thoroughly combine the oat milk, applesauce, vanilla, salt, nutmeg, cloves and cinnamon.
- ❖ Dip each slice of bread into the custard mixture until well coated on all sides.
- ❖ Preheat the coconut oil in a frying pan over medium-high heat. Cook for about 3 minutes on each side, until golden brown.
- ❖ Drizzle the French toast with maple syrup and serve immediately. Enjoy

15) NUTTY BREAKFAST BREAD PUDDING

Preparation Time: 2 hours 10 minutes

Servings: 6

Ingredients:

- ✓ 1 ½ cups almond milk
- ✓ 1/2 cup maple syrup
- ✓ 2 tbsp almond butter
- ✓ 1/2 tsp vanilla extract
- ✓ 1/2 tsp almond extract
- ✓ 1/2 tsp ground cinnamon
- ✓ 1/2 tsp ground cloves
- ✓ 1/3 tsp kosher salt
- ✓ 1/2 cup almonds, roughly chopped
- ✓ 4 cups day-old white bread, cubed

Directions:

- ❖ In a mixing bowl, combine the almond milk, maple syrup, almond butter, vanilla extract, almond extract and spices.
- ❖ Add the bread cubes to the custard mixture and stir to combine well. Fold in the almonds and allow it to rest for about 1 hour.
- ❖ Then, spoon the mixture into a lightly oiled casserole dish.
- ❖ Bake in the preheated oven at 350 degrees F for about 1 hour or until the top is golden brown.
- ❖ Place the bread pudding on a wire rack for 10 minutes before slicing and serving. Enjoy

16) OMELETTE WITH MUSHROOMS AND PEPPERS

Preparation Time: 30 minutes

Servings: 4

Ingredients:

- ✓ 4 tbsp olive oil
- ✓ 1 red onion, minced
- ✓ 1 red bell pepper, sliced
- ✓ 1 tsp garlic, finely chopped
- ✓ 1 pound button mushrooms, sliced
- ✓ Sea salt and ground black pepper, to taste
- ✓ 1/2 tsp dried oregano
- ✓ 1/2 tsp dried dill
- ✓ 16 ounces tofu, drained and crumbled
- ✓ 2 tbsp nutritional yeast
- ✓ 1/2 tsp turmeric powder
- ✓ 4 tbsp corn flour
- ✓ 1/3 cup oat milk, unsweetened

Directions:

- ❖ Preheat 2 tbsp of the olive oil in a nonstick skillet over medium-high heat. Then, cook the onion and pepper for about 4 minutes until tender and fragrant.
- ❖ Add in the garlic and mushrooms and continue to sauté an additional 2 to 3 minutes or until aromatic. Season with salt, black pepper, oregano and dill. Reserve.
- ❖ In your blender or food processor, mix the tofu, nutritional yeast, turmeric powder, corn flour and milk. Process until you have a smooth and uniform paste.
- ❖ In the same skillet, heat 1 tbsp of the olive oil until sizzling. Pour in 1/2 of the tofu mixture and spread it with a spatula.
- ❖ Cook for about 6 minutes or until set; flip and cook it for another 3 minutes. Slide the omelet onto a serving plate.
- ❖ Spoon 1/2 of the mushroom filling over half of the omelet. Fold the unfilled half of omelet over the filling.
- ❖ Repeat with another omelet. Cut them into halves and serve warm. Enjoy

17) COLD HEMP AND BLACKBERRY SMOOTHIE BOWL

Preparation Time: 10 minutes

Servings: 2

Ingredients:

- ✓ 2 tbsp hemp seeds
- ✓ 1/2 cup coconut milk
- ✓ 1 cup coconut yogurt
- ✓ 1 cup blackberries, frozen
- ✓ 2 small-sized bananas, frozen
- ✓ 4 tbsp granola

Directions:

- ❖ In your blender, mix all ingredients, trying to keep the liquids at the bottom of the blender to help it break up the fruits.
- ❖ Divide your smoothie between serving bowls.
- ❖ Garnish each bowl with granola and some extra frozen berries, if desired. Serve immediately

18) CHOCOLATE AND WALNUT STEEL-CUT OATS

Preparation Time: 30 minutes

Servings: 3

Ingredients:

- ✓ 2 cups oat milk
- ✓ 1/3 cup steel-cut oats
- ✓ 1 tbsp coconut oil
- ✓ 1/4 cup coconut sugar
- ✓ A pinch of grated nutmeg
- ✓ A pinch of flaky sea salt
- ✓ 1/4 tsp cinnamon powder
- ✓ 1/4 tsp vanilla extract
- ✓ 4 tbsp cocoa powder
- ✓ 1/3 cup English walnut halves
- ✓ 4 tbsp chocolate chips

Directions:

- ❖ Bring the oat milk and oats to a boil over a moderately high heat. Then, turn the heat to low and add in the coconut oil, sugar and spices; let it simmer for about 25 minutes, stirring periodically.
- ❖ Add in the cocoa powder and continue simmering an additional 3 minutes.
- ❖ Spoon the oatmeal into serving bowls. Top each bowl with the walnut halves and chocolate chips.
- ❖ Enjoy

19) BUCKWHEAT PORRIDGE WITH APPLES-ALMONDS

Preparation Time: 20 minutes

Servings: 3

Ingredients:

- ✓ 1 cup buckwheat groats, toasted
- ✓ 3/4 cup water
- ✓ 1 cup rice milk
- ✓ 1/4 tsp sea salt
- ✓ 3 tbsp agave syrup
- ✓ 1 cup apples, cored and diced
- ✓ 3 tbsp almonds, slivered
- ✓ 2 tbsp coconut flakes
- ✓ 2 tbsp hemp seeds

Directions:

- ❖ In a saucepan, bring the buckwheat groats, water, milk and salt to a boil. Immediately turn the heat to a simmer; let it simmer for about 13 minutes until it has softened. Stir in the agave syrup. Divide the porridge between three serving bowls.
- ❖ Garnish each serving with the apples, almonds, coconut and hemp seeds. Enjoy

20) ORIGINAL SPANISH TORTILLA

Preparation Time: 35 minutes

Servings: 2

Ingredients:

- ✓ 3 tbsp olive oil
- ✓ 2 medium potatoes, peeled and diced
- ✓ 1/2 white onion, chopped
- ✓ 8 tbsp gram flour
- ✓ 8 tbsp water
- ✓ Sea salt and ground black pepper, to season
- ✓ 1/2 tsp Spanish paprika

Directions:

- ❖ Heat 2 tbsp of the olive oil in a frying pan over a moderate flame. Now, cook the potatoes and onion; cook for about 20 minutes or until tender; reserve.
- ❖ In a mixing bowl, thoroughly combine the flour, water, salt, black pepper and paprika. Add in the potato/onion mixture.
- ❖ Heat the remaining 1 tbsp of the olive oil in the same frying pan. Pour 1/2 of the batter into the frying pan. Cook your tortilla for about 11 minutes, turning it once or twice to promote even cooking.
- ❖ Repeat with the remaining batter and serve warm

21) CHOCOLATE AND MANGO QUINOA BOWL

Preparation Time: 35 minutes

Servings: 2

Ingredients:

- ✓ 1 cup quinoa
- ✓ 1 tsp ground cinnamon
- ✓ 1 cup non-dairy milk
- ✓ 1 large mango, chopped
- ✓ 3 tbsp unsweetened cocoa powder
- ✓ 2 tbsp almond butter
- ✓ 1 tbsp hemp seeds
- ✓ 1 tbsp walnuts
- ✓ ¼ cup raspberries

Directions:

- ❖ In a pot, combine the quinoa, cinnamon, milk, and 1 cup of water over medium heat. Bring to a boil, low heat, and simmer covered for 25-30 minutes. In a bowl, mash the mango and mix cocoa powder, almond butter, and hemp seeds. In a serving bowl, place cooked quinoa and mango mixture.
- ❖ Top with walnuts and raspberries. Serve immediately

22) ORANGE AND CARROT MUFFINS WITH CHERRIES

Preparation Time: 45 minutes

Servings: 6

Ingredients:

- ✓ 1 tsp vegetable oil
- ✓ 2 tbsp almond butter
- ✓ ¼ cup non-dairy milk
- ✓ 1 orange, peeled
- ✓ 1 carrot, coarsely chopped
- ✓ 2 tbsp chopped dried cherries
- ✓ 3 tbsp molasses
- ✓ 2 tbsp ground flaxseed
- ✓ 1 tsp apple cider vinegar
- ✓ 1 tsp pure vanilla extract
- ✓ ½ tsp ground cinnamon
- ✓ ½ tsp ground ginger
- ✓ ¼ tsp ground nutmeg
- ✓ ¼ tsp allspice
- ✓ ¾ cup whole-wheat flour
- ✓ 1 tsp baking powder
- ✓ ½ tsp baking soda
- ✓ ½ cup rolled oats
- ✓ 2 tbsp raisins
- ✓ 2 tbsp sunflower seeds

Directions:

- ❖ Preheat oven to 350 F. Grease 6 muffin cups with vegetable oil.
- ❖ In a food processor, add the almond butter, milk, orange, carrot, cherries, molasses, flaxseed, vinegar, vanilla, cinnamon, ginger, nutmeg, and allspice and blend until smooth.
- ❖ In a bowl, combine the flour, baking powder, and baking soda. Fold in the wet mixture and gently stir to combine. Mix in the oats, raisins, and sunflower seeds. Divide the batter between muffin cups. Put in a baking tray and bake for 30 minutes

23) QUINOA LEMONY MUFFINS

Preparation Time: 25 minutes

Servings: 5

Ingredients:

- ✓ 2 tbsp coconut oil melted, plus more for coating the muffin tin
- ✓ ¼ cup ground flaxseed
- ✓ 2 cups unsweetened lemon curd
- ✓ ½ cup pure date sugar
- ✓ 1 tsp apple cider vinegar
- ✓ 2 ½ cups whole-wheat flour
- ✓ 1 ½ cups cooked quinoa
- ✓ 2 tsp baking soda
- ✓ A pinch of salt
- ✓ ½ cup raisins

Directions:

- ❖ Preheat oven to 400 F.
- ❖ In a bowl, combine the flaxseed and ½ cup water. Stir in the lemon curd, sugar, coconut oil, and vinegar. Add in flour, quinoa, baking soda, and salt. Put in the raisins, be careful not too fluffy.
- ❖ Divide the batter between greased with coconut oil cups of the tin and bake for 20 minutes until golden and set. Allow cooling slightly before removing it from the tin. Serve

24) OATMEAL ALMOND PORRIDGE

Preparation Time: 25 minutes

Servings: 4

Ingredients:

- ✓ 2 ½ cups vegetable broth
- ✓ 2 ½ cups almond milk
- ✓ ½ cup steel-cut oats
- ✓ 1 tbsp pearl barley
- ✓ ½ cup slivered almonds
- ✓ ¼ cup nutritional yeast
- ✓ 2 cups old-fashioned rolled oats

Directions:

- ❖ • Pour the broth and almond milk in a pot over medium heat and bring to a boil. Stir in oats, pearl barley, almond slivers, and nutritional yeast. Reduce the heat and simmer for 20 minutes. Add in the rolled oats, cook for an additional 5 minutes, until creamy. Allow cooling before serving

25) BREAKFAST PECAN AND PEAR FARRO

Preparation Time: 20 minutes

Servings: 4

Ingredients:

- ✓ 2 cups water
- ✓ ½ tsp salt
- ✓ 1 cup farro
- ✓ 1 tbsp plant butter
- ✓ 2 pears, peeled, cored, and chopped
- ✓ ¼ cup chopped pecans

Directions:

- ❖ Bring water to a boil in a pot over high heat. Stir in salt and farro. Lower the heat, cover, and simmer for 15 minutes until the farro is tender and the liquid has absorbed. Turn the heat off and add in the butter, pears, and pecans. Cover and rest for 12-15 minutes.
- ❖ Serve immediately

26) BLACKBERRY WAFFLES

Preparation Time: 15 minutes

Servings: 4

Ingredients:

- ✓ 1 ½ cups whole-heat flour
- ✓ ½ cup old-fashioned oats
- ✓ ¼ cup date sugar
- ✓ 3 tsp baking powder
- ✓ ½ tsp salt
- ✓ 1 tsp ground cinnamon
- ✓ 2 cups soy milk
- ✓ 1 tbsp fresh lemon juice
- ✓ 1 tsp lemon zest
- ✓ ¼ cup plant butter, melted
- ✓ ½ cup fresh blackberries

Directions:

- ❖ Preheat the waffle iron.
- ❖ In a bowl, mix flour, oats, sugar, baking powder, salt, and cinnamon. Set aside. In another bowl, combine milk, lemon juice, lemon zest, and butter. Pour into the wet ingredients and whisk to combine. Add the batter to the hot greased waffle iron, using approximately a ladleful for each waffle. Cook for 3-5 minutes, until golden brown. Repeat the process until no batter is left.
- ❖ Serve topped with blackberries

27) ORIGINAL WALNUT WAFFLES WITH MAPLE SYRUP

Preparation Time: 15 minutes

Servings: 4

Ingredients:

- ✓ 1 ¾ cups whole-wheat flour
- ✓ ⅓ cup coarsely ground walnuts
- ✓ 1 tbsp baking powder
- ✓ 1 ½p cups soy milk
- ✓ 3 tbsp pure maple syrup
- ✓ 3 tbsp plant butter, melted

Directions:

- ❖ Preheat the waffle iron and grease with oil. Combine the flour, walnuts, baking powder, and salt in a bowl. Set aside. In another bowl, mix the milk and butter. Pour into the walnut mixture and whisk until well combined. Spoon a ladleful of the batter onto the waffle iron.
- ❖ Cook for 3-5 minutes, until golden brown. Repeat the process until no batter is left. Top with maple syrup to serve

28) ORANGE AND BRAN CUPS WITH DATES

Preparation Time: 30 minutes

Servings: 12

Ingredients:

- ✓ 1 tsp vegetable oil
- ✓ 3 cups bran flakes cereal
- ✓ 1 ½ cups whole-wheat flour
- ✓ ½ cup dates, chopped
- ✓ 3 tsp baking powder
- ✓ ½ tsp ground cinnamon
- ✓ ½ tsp salt
- ✓ ⅓ cup brown sugar
- ✓ ¾ cup fresh orange juice

Directions:

- ❖ Preheat oven to 400 F. Grease a 12-cup muffin tin with oil.
- ❖ Mix the bran flakes, flour, dates, baking powder, cinnamon, and salt in a bowl. In another bowl, combine the sugar and orange juice until blended. Pour into the dry mixture and whisk. Divide the mixture between the cups of the muffin tin. Bake for 20 minutes or until golden brown and set. Cool for a few minutes before removing from the tin and serve

29) MACADAMIA NUTS AND APPLE-DATE COUSCOUS

Preparation Time: 20 minutes

Servings: 4

Ingredients:

- ✓ 3 cups apple juice
- ✓ 1 ½ cups couscous
- ✓ 1 tsp ground cinnamon
- ✓ ¼ tsp ground cloves
- ✓ ½ cup dried dates
- ✓ ½ cup chopped macadamia nuts

Directions:

- ❖ Pour the apple juice into a pot over medium heat and bring to a boil. Stir in couscous, cinnamon, and cloves. Turn the heat off and cover. Let sit for 5 minutes until the liquid is absorbed.
- ❖ Using a fork, fluff the couscous and add the dates and macadamia nuts, stir to combine. Serve warm

30) BLUEBERRY COCONUT MUFFINS

Preparation Time: 30 minutes

Servings: 12

Ingredients:

- ✓ 1 tbsp coconut oil melted
- ✓ 1 cup quick-cooking oats
- ✓ 1 cup boiling water
- ✓ ½ cup almond milk
- ✓ ¼ cup ground flaxseed
- ✓ 1 tsp almond extract
- ✓ 1 tsp apple cider vinegar
- ✓ 1 ½ cups whole-wheat flour
- ✓ ½ cup pure date sugar
- ✓ 2 tsp baking soda
- ✓ A pinch of salt
- ✓ 1 cup blueberries

Directions:

- ❖ Preheat oven to 400 F.
- ❖ In a bowl, stir in the oats with boiling water until they are softened. Pour in the coconut oil, milk, flaxseed, almond extract, and vinegar. Add in the flour, sugar, baking soda, and salt. Gently stir in blueberries.
- ❖ Divide the batter between a greased with coconut oil muffin tin. Bake for 20 minutes until lightly brown. Allow cooling for 10 minutes. Using a spatula, run the sides of the muffins to take out. Serve

31) SWISS CHARD SCRAMBLED TOFU

Preparation Time: 35 minutes

Servings: 5

Ingredients:

- ✓ 1 (14-oz) package tofu, crumbled
- ✓ 2 tsp olive oil
- ✓ 1 onion, chopped
- ✓ 3 cloves minced garlic
- ✓ 1 celery stalk, chopped
- ✓ 2 large carrots, chopped
- ✓ 1 tsp chili powder
- ✓ ½ tsp ground cumin
- ✓ ½ tsp ground turmeric
- ✓ Salt and black pepper to taste
- ✓ 5 cups Swiss chard

Directions:

- ❖ Heat the oil in a skillet over medium heat. Add in the onion, garlic, celery, and carrots. Sauté for 5 minutes. Stir in tofu, chili powder, cumin, turmeric, salt, and pepper, cook for 7-8 minutes more.
- ❖ Mix in the Swiss chard and cook until wilted, about 3 minutes. Allow cooling and seal and serve

32) BANANA TANGERINE TOAST

Preparation Time: 25 minutes

Servings: 4

Ingredients:

- ✓ 3 bananas
- ✓ 1 cup almond milk
- ✓ Zest and juice of 1 tangerine
- ✓ 1 tsp ground cinnamon
- ✓ ¼ tsp grated nutmeg
- ✓ 4 slices bread
- ✓ 1 tbsp olive oil

Directions:

- ❖ Blend the bananas, almond milk, tangerine juice, tangerine zest, cinnamon, and nutmeg until smooth in a food processor. Spread into a baking dish. Submerge the bread slices in the mixture for 3-4 minutes.
- ❖ Heat the oil in a skillet over medium heat. Fry the bread for 5 minutes until golden brown. Serve hot

33) MAPLE BANANA OATS

Preparation Time: 35 minutes

Servings: 4

Ingredients:

- ✓ 3 cups water
- ✓ 1 cup steel-cut oats
- ✓ 2 bananas, mashed
- ✓ ¼ cup pumpkin seeds
- ✓ 2 tbsp maple syrup
- ✓ A pinch of salt

Directions:

- ❖ Bring water to a boil in a pot, add in oats, and lower the heat. Cook for 20-30 minutes. Put in the mashed bananas, cook for 3-5 minutes more. Stir in maple syrup, pumpkin seeds, and salt. Serve

34) GINGERBREAD BELGIAN WAFFLES

Preparation Time: 25 minutes

Servings: 3

Ingredients:

- ✓ 1 cup all-purpose flour
- ✓ 1 tsp baking powder
- ✓ 1 tbsp brown sugar
- ✓ 1 tsp ground ginger
- ✓ 1 cup almond milk
- ✓ 1 tsp vanilla extract
- ✓ 2 olive oil

Directions:

- ❖ Preheat a waffle iron according to the manufacturer's instructions.
- ❖ In a mixing bowl, thoroughly combine the flour, baking powder, brown sugar, ground ginger, almond milk, vanilla extract and olive oil.
- ❖ Beat until everything is well blended.
- ❖ Ladle 1/3 of the batter into the preheated waffle iron and cook until the waffles are golden and crisp. Repeat with the remaining batter.
- ❖ Serve your waffles with blackberry jam, if desired. Enjoy

35) BANANA AND WALNUTS PORRIDGE

Preparation Time: 15 minutes

Servings: 4

Ingredients:

- ✓ 1 cup rolled oats
- ✓ 1 cup spelt flakes
- ✓ 2 cups unsweetened almond milk
- ✓ 4 tbsp agave nectar
- ✓ 4 tbsp walnuts, chopped
- ✓ 2 bananas, sliced

Directions:

- ❖ In a nonstick skillet, fry the oats and spelt flakes until fragrant, working in batches.
- ❖ Bring the milk to a boil and add in the oats, spelt flakes and agave nectar.
- ❖ Turn the heat to a simmer and let it cook for 6 to 7 minutes, stirring occasionally. Top with walnuts and bananas and serve warm. Enjoy

SOUPS, STEW AND SALADS

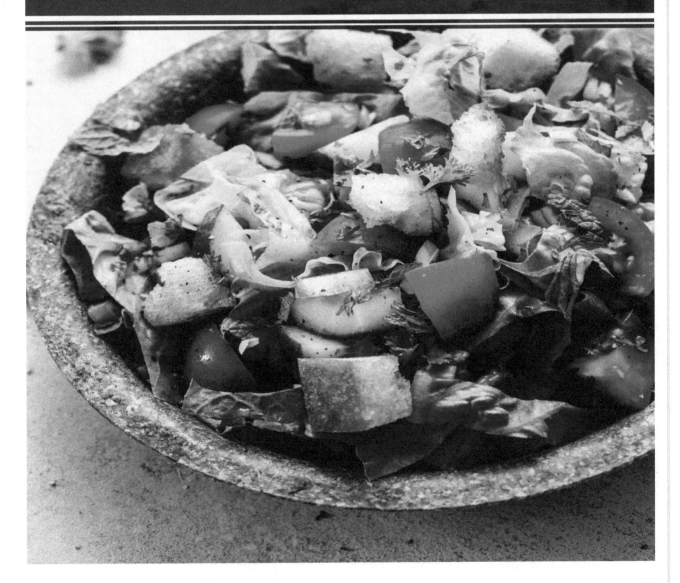

36) BLACK BEAN QUINOA SALAD

Preparation Time: 15 minutes + chilling time

Servings: 4

Ingredients:

- ✓ 2 cups water
- ✓ 1 cup quinoa, rinsed
- ✓ 16 ounces canned black beans, drained
- ✓ 2 Roma tomatoes, sliced
- ✓ 1 red onion, thinly sliced
- ✓ 1 cucumber, seeded and chopped
- ✓ 2 cloves garlic, pressed or minced
- ✓ 2 Italian peppers, seeded and sliced
- ✓ 2 tbsp fresh parsley, chopped
- ✓ 2 tbsp fresh cilantro, chopped
- ✓ 1/4 cup olive oil
- ✓ 1 lemon, freshly squeezed
- ✓ 1 tbsp apple cider vinegar
- ✓ 1/2 tsp dried dill weed
- ✓ 1/2 tsp dried oregano
- ✓ Sea salt and ground black pepper, to taste

Directions:

- ❖ Place the water and quinoa in a saucepan and bring it to a rolling boil. Immediately turn the heat to a simmer.
- ❖ Let it simmer for about 13 minutes until the quinoa has absorbed all of the water; fluff the quinoa with a fork and let it cool completely. Then, transfer the quinoa to a salad bowl.
- ❖ Add the remaining ingredients to the salad bowl and toss to combine well. Enjoy

37) POWER BULGUR SALAD WITH HERBS

Preparation Time: 20 minutes + chilling time

Servings: 4

Ingredients:

- ✓ 2 cups water
- ✓ 1 cup bulgur
- ✓ 12 ounces canned chickpeas, drained
- ✓ 1 Persian cucumber, thinly sliced
- ✓ 2 bell peppers, seeded and thinly sliced
- ✓ 1 jalapeno pepper, seeded and thinly sliced
- ✓ 2 Roma tomatoes, sliced
- ✓ 1 onion, thinly sliced
- ✓ 2 tbsp fresh basil, chopped
- ✓ 2 tbsp fresh parsley, chopped
- ✓ 2 tbsp fresh mint, chopped
- ✓ 2 tbsp fresh chives, chopped
- ✓ 4 tbsp olive oil
- ✓ 1 tbsp balsamic vinegar
- ✓ 1 tbsp lemon juice
- ✓ 1 tsp fresh garlic, pressed
- ✓ Sea salt and freshly ground black pepper, to taste
- ✓ 2 tbsp nutritional yeast
- ✓ 1/2 cup Kalamata olives, sliced

Directions:

- ❖ In a saucepan, bring the water and bulgur to a boil. Immediately turn the heat to a simmer and let it cook for about 20 minutes or until the bulgur is tender and water is almost absorbed. Fluff with a fork and spread on a large tray to let cool.
- ❖ Place the bulgur in a salad bowl followed by the chickpeas, cucumber, peppers, tomatoes, onion, basil, parsley, mint and chives.
- ❖ In a small mixing dish, whisk the olive oil, balsamic vinegar, lemon juice, garlic, salt and black pepper. Dress the salad and toss to combine.
- ❖ Sprinkle nutritional yeast over the top, garnish with olives and serve at room temperature. Enjoy

38) ORIGINAL ROASTED PEPPER SALAD

Preparation Time: 15 minutes + chilling time

Servings: 3

Ingredients:

- ✓ 6 bell peppers
- ✓ 3 tbsp extra-virgin olive oil
- ✓ 3 tsp red wine vinegar
- ✓ 3 garlic cloves, finely chopped
- ✓ 2 tbsp fresh parsley, chopped
- ✓ Sea salt and freshly cracked black pepper, to taste
- ✓ 1/2 tsp red pepper flakes
- ✓ 6 tbsp pine nuts, roughly chopped

Directions:

- ❖ Broil the peppers on a parchment-lined baking sheet for about 10 minutes, rotating the pan halfway through the cooking time, until they are charred on all sides.
- ❖ Then, cover the peppers with a plastic wrap to steam. Discard the skin, seeds and cores.
- ❖ Slice the peppers into strips and toss them with the remaining ingredients. Place in your refrigerator until ready to serve. Enjoy

39) WINTER HEARTY QUINOA SOUP

Preparation Time: 25 minutes   **Servings: 4**

Ingredients:

- 2 tbsp olive oil
- 1 onion, chopped
- 2 carrots, peeled and chopped
- 1 parsnip, chopped
- 1 celery stalk, chopped
- 1 cup yellow squash, chopped
- 4 garlic cloves, pressed or minced
- 4 cups roasted vegetable broth
- 2 medium tomatoes, crushed
- 1 cup quinoa
- Sea salt and ground black pepper, to taste
- 1 bay laurel
- 2 cup Swiss chard, tough ribs removed and torn into pieces
- 2 tbsp Italian parsley, chopped

Directions:

- ❖ In a heavy-bottomed pot, heat the olive over medium-high heat. Now, sauté the onion, carrot, parsnip, celery and yellow squash for about 3 minutes or until the vegetables are just tender.
- ❖ Add in the garlic and continue to sauté for 1 minute or until aromatic.
- ❖ Then, stir in the vegetable broth, tomatoes, quinoa, salt, pepper and bay laurel; bring to a boil. Immediately reduce the heat to a simmer and let it cook for 13 minutes.
- ❖ Fold in the Swiss chard; continue to simmer until the chard wilts.
- ❖ Ladle into individual bowls and serve garnished with the fresh parsley. Enjoy

40) GREEN LENTIL SALAD

Preparation Time: 20 minutes + chilling time   **Servings: 5**

Ingredients:

- 1 ½ cups green lentils, rinsed
- 2 cups arugula
- 2 cups Romaine lettuce, torn into pieces
- 1 cup baby spinach
- 1/4 cup fresh basil, chopped
- 1/2 cup shallots, chopped
- 2 garlic cloves, finely chopped
- 1/4 cup oil-packed sun-dried tomatoes, rinsed and chopped
- 5 tbsp extra-virgin olive oil
- 3 tbsp fresh lemon juice
- Sea salt and ground black pepper, to taste

Directions:

- ❖ In a large-sized saucepan, bring 4 ½ cups of the water and red lentils to a boil.
- ❖ Immediately turn the heat to a simmer and continue to cook your lentils for a further 15 to 17 minutes or until they've softened but not mushy. Drain and let it cool completely.
- ❖ Transfer the lentils to a salad bowl; toss the lentils with the remaining ingredients until well combined.
- ❖ Serve chilled or at room temperature. Enjoy

41) CHICKPEA, ACORN SQUASH, AND COUSCOUS SOUP

Preparation Time: 20 minutes   **Servings: 4**

Ingredients:

- 2 tbsp olive oil
- 1 shallot, chopped
- 1 carrot, trimmed and chopped
- 2 cups acorn squash, chopped
- 1 stalk celery, chopped
- 1 tsp garlic, finely chopped
- 1 tsp dried rosemary, chopped
- 1 tsp dried thyme, chopped
- 2 cups cream of onion soup
- 2 cups water
- 1 cup dry couscous
- Sea salt and ground black pepper, to taste
- 1/2 tsp red pepper flakes
- 6 ounces canned chickpeas, drained
- 2 tbsp fresh lemon juice

Directions:

- ❖ In a heavy-bottomed pot, heat the olive over medium-high heat. Now, sauté the shallot, carrot, acorn squash and celery for about 3 minutes or until the vegetables are just tender.
- ❖ Add in the garlic, rosemary and thyme and continue to sauté for 1 minute or until aromatic.
- ❖ Then, stir in the soup, water, couscous, salt, black pepper and red pepper flakes; bring to a boil. Immediately reduce the heat to a simmer and let it cook for 12 minutes.
- ❖ Fold in the canned chickpeas; continue to simmer until heated through or about 5 minutes more.
- ❖ Ladle into individual bowls and drizzle with the lemon juice over the top. Enjoy

42) GARLIC CROSTINI WITH CABBAGE SOUP

Preparation Time: 1 hour   **Servings: 4**

Ingredients:

- ✓ Soup:
- ✓ 2 tbsp olive oil
- ✓ 1 medium leek, chopped
- ✓ 1 cup turnip, chopped
- ✓ 1 parsnip, chopped
- ✓ 1 carrot, chopped
- ✓ 2 cups cabbage, shredded
- ✓ 2 garlic cloves, finely chopped
- ✓ 4 cups vegetable broth
- ✓ 2 bay leaves
- ✓ Sea salt and ground black pepper, to taste
- ✓ 1/4 tsp cumin seeds
- ✓ 1/2 tsp mustard seeds
- ✓ 1 tsp dried basil
- ✓ 2 tomatoes, pureed
- ✓ Crostini:
- ✓ 8 slices of baguette
- ✓ 2 heads garlic
- ✓ 4 tbsp extra-virgin olive oil

Directions:

- ❖ In a soup pot, heat 2 tbsp of the olive over medium-high heat. Now, sauté the leek, turnip, parsnip and carrot for about 4 minutes or until the vegetables are crisp-tender.
- ❖ Add in the garlic and cabbage and continue to sauté for 1 minute or until aromatic.
- ❖ Then, stir in the vegetable broth, bay leaves, salt, black pepper, cumin seeds, mustard seeds, dried basil and pureed tomatoes; bring to a boil. Immediately reduce the heat to a simmer and let it cook for about 20 minutes.
- ❖ Meanwhile, preheat your oven to 375 degrees F. Now, roast the garlic and baguette slices for about 15 minutes. Remove the crostini from the oven.
- ❖ Continue baking the garlic for 45 minutes more or until very tender. Allow the garlic to cool.
- ❖ Now, cut each head of the garlic using a sharp serrated knife in order to separate all the cloves.
- ❖ Squeeze the roasted garlic cloves out of their skins. Mash the garlic pulp with 4 tbsp of the extra-virgin olive oil.
- ❖ Spread the roasted garlic mixture evenly on the tops of the crostini. Serve with the warm soup. Enjoy

43) GREEN BEAN SOUP CREAM

Preparation Time: 35 minutes   **Servings: 4**

Ingredients:

- ✓ 1 tbsp sesame oil
- ✓ 1 onion, chopped
- ✓ 1 green pepper, seeded and chopped
- ✓ 2 russet potatoes, peeled and diced
- ✓ 2 garlic cloves, chopped
- ✓ 4 cups vegetable broth
- ✓ 1 pound green beans, trimmed
- ✓ Sea salt and ground black pepper, to season
- ✓ 1 cup full-fat coconut milk

Directions:

- ❖ In a heavy-bottomed pot, heat the sesame over medium-high heat. Now, sauté the onion, peppers and potatoes for about 5 minutes, stirring periodically.
- ❖ Add in the garlic and continue sautéing for 1 minute or until fragrant.
- ❖ Then, stir in the vegetable broth, green beans, salt and black pepper; bring to a boil. Immediately reduce the heat to a simmer and let it cook for 20 minutes.
- ❖ Puree the green bean mixture using an immersion blender until creamy and uniform.
- ❖ Return the pureed mixture to the pot. Fold in the coconut milk and continue to simmer until heated through or about 5 minutes longer.
- ❖ Ladle into individual bowls and serve hot. Enjoy

44) FRENCH TRADITIONAL ONION SOUP

Preparation Time: 1 hour 30 minutes   **Servings: 4**

Ingredients:

- ✓ 2 tbsp olive oil
- ✓ 2 large yellow onions, thinly sliced
- ✓ 2 thyme sprigs, chopped
- ✓ 2 rosemary sprigs, chopped
- ✓ 2 tsp balsamic vinegar
- ✓ 4 cups vegetable stock
- ✓ Sea salt and ground black pepper, to taste

Directions:

- ❖ In a or Dutch oven, heat the olive oil over a moderate heat. Now, cook the onions with thyme, rosemary and 1 tsp of the sea salt for about 2 minutes.
- ❖ Now, turn the heat to medium-low and continue cooking until the onions caramelize or about 50 minutes.
- ❖ Add in the balsamic vinegar and continue to cook for a further 15 more. Add in the stock, salt and black pepper and continue simmering for 20 to 25 minutes.
- ❖ Serve with toasted bread and enjoy

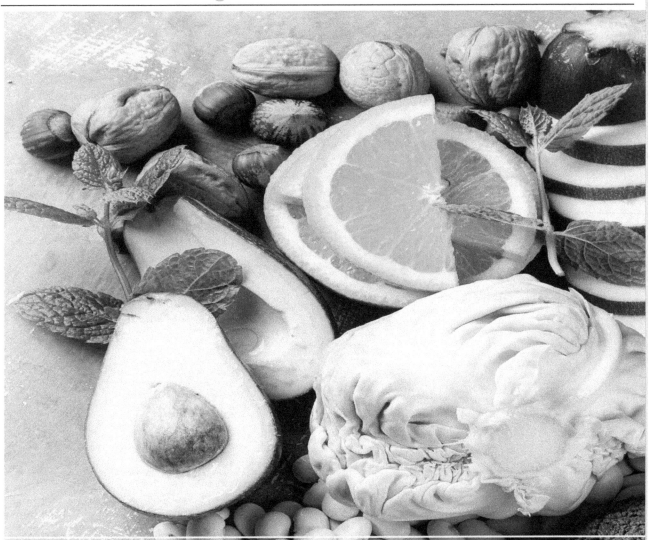

VEGETABLES AND SIDE DISHES

45) ROASTED ASPARAGUS WITH SESAME SEEDS

Preparation Time: 25 minutes

Servings: 4

Ingredients:

- ✓ 1 ½ pounds asparagus, trimmed
- ✓ 4 tbsp extra-virgin olive oil
- ✓ Sea salt and ground black pepper, to taste
- ✓ 1/2 tsp dried oregano

- ✓ 1/2 tsp dried basil
- ✓ 1 tsp red pepper flakes, crushed
- ✓ 4 tbsp sesame seeds
- ✓ 2 tbsp fresh chives, roughly chopped

Directions:

- ❖ Start by preheating the oven to 400 degrees F. Then, line a baking sheet with parchment paper.
- ❖ Toss the asparagus with the olive oil, salt, black pepper, oregano, basil and red pepper flakes. Now, arrange your asparagus in a single layer on the prepared baking sheet.
- ❖ Roast your asparagus for approximately 20 minutes.
- ❖ Sprinkle sesame seeds over your asparagus and continue to bake an additional 5 minutes or until the asparagus spears are crisp-tender and the sesame seeds are lightly toasted.
- ❖ Garnish with fresh chives and serve warm. Enjoy

46) GREEK-STYLE EGGPLANT SKILLET

Preparation Time: 15 minutes

Servings: 4

Ingredients:

- ✓ 4 tbsp olive oil
- ✓ 1 ½ pounds eggplant, peeled and sliced
- ✓ 1 tsp garlic, minced
- ✓ 1 tomato, crushed
- ✓ Sea salt and ground black pepper, to taste

- ✓ 1 tsp cayenne pepper
- ✓ 1/2 tsp dried oregano
- ✓ 1/4 tsp ground bay leaf
- ✓ 2 ounces Kalamata olives, pitted and sliced

Directions:

- ❖ Heat the oil in a sauté pan over medium-high flame.
- ❖ Then, sauté the eggplant for about 9 minutes or until just tender.
- ❖ Add in the remaining ingredients, cover and continue to cook for 2 to 3 minutes more or until thoroughly cooked. Serve warm

47) CAULIFLOWER RICE

Preparation Time: 10 minutes

Servings: 5

Ingredients:

- ✓ 2 medium heads cauliflower, stems and leaves removed
- ✓ 4 tbsp extra-virgin olive oil
- ✓ 4 garlic cloves, pressed

- ✓ 1/2 tsp red pepper flakes, crushed
- ✓ Sea salt and ground black pepper, to taste
- ✓ 1/4 cup flat-leaf parsley, roughly chopped

Directions:

- ❖ Pulse the cauliflower in a food processor with the S-blade until they're broken into "rice".
- ❖ Heat the olive oil in a saucepan over medium-high heat. Once hot, cook the garlic until fragrant or about 1 minute.
- ❖ Add in the cauliflower rice, red pepper, salt and black pepper and continue sautéing for a further 7 to 8 minutes.
- ❖ Taste, adjust the seasonings and garnish with fresh parsley. Enjoy

48) GARLICKY KALE

Preparation Time: 10 minutes

Servings: 4

Ingredients:

- ✓ 4 tbsp olive oil
- ✓ 4 cloves garlic, chopped
- ✓ 1 ½ pounds fresh kale, tough stems and ribs removed, torn into pieces
- ✓ 1 cup vegetable broth

- ✓ 1/2 tsp cumin seeds
- ✓ 1/2 tsp dried oregano
- ✓ 1/2 tsp paprika
- ✓ 1 tsp onion powder
- ✓ Sea salt and ground black pepper, to taste

Directions:

- ❖ In a saucepan, heat the olive oil over a moderately high heat. Now, sauté the garlic for about 1 minute or until aromatic.
- ❖ Add in the kale in batches, gradually adding the vegetable broth; stir to promote even cooking.
- ❖ Turn the heat to a simmer, add in the spices and let it cook for 5 to 6 minutes, until the kale leaves wilt.
- ❖ Serve warm and enjoy

49) ARTICHOKES BRAISED IN LEMON AND OLIVE OIL

Preparation Time: 35 minutes

Servings: 4

Ingredients:

- ✓ 1 ½ cups water
- ✓ 2 lemons, freshly squeezed
- ✓ 2 pounds artichokes, trimmed, tough outer leaves and chokes removed
- ✓ 1 handful fresh Italian parsley
- ✓ 2 thyme sprigs
- ✓ 2 rosemary sprigs
- ✓ 2 bay leaves
- ✓ 2 garlic cloves, chopped
- ✓ 1/3 cup olive oil
- ✓ Sea salt and ground black pepper, to taste
- ✓ 1/2 tsp red pepper flakes

Directions:

- ❖ Fill a bowl with water and add in the lemon juice. Place the cleaned artichokes in the bowl, keeping them completely submerged.
- ❖ In another small bowl, thoroughly combine the herbs and garlic. Rub your artichokes with the herb mixture.
- ❖ Pour the lemon water and olive oil in a saucepan; add the artichokes to the saucepan. Turn the heat to a simmer and continue to cook, covered, for about 30 minutes until the artichokes are crisp-tender.
- ❖ To serve, drizzle the artichokes with cooking juices, season them with the salt, black pepper and red pepper flakes. Enjoy

50) ROSEMARY AND GARLIC ROASTED CARROTS

Preparation Time: 25 minutes

Servings: 4

Ingredients:

- ✓ 2 pounds carrots, trimmed and halved lengthwise
- ✓ 4 tbsp olive oil
- ✓ 2 tbsp champagne vinegar
- ✓ 4 cloves garlic, minced
- ✓ 2 sprigs rosemary, chopped
- ✓ Sea salt and ground black pepper, to taste
- ✓ 4 tbsp pine nuts, chopped

Directions:

- ❖ Begin by preheating your oven to 400 degrees F.
- ❖ Toss the carrots with the olive oil, vinegar, garlic, rosemary, salt and black pepper. Arrange them in a single layer on a parchment-lined roasting sheet.
- ❖ Roast the carrots in the preheated oven for about 20 minutes, until fork-tender.
- ❖ Garnish the carrots with the pine nuts and serve immediately. Enjoy

51) MEDITERRANEAN-STYLE GREEN BEANS

Preparation Time: 20 minutes

Servings: 4

Ingredients:

- ✓ 2 tbsp olive oil
- ✓ 1 red bell pepper, seeded and diced
- ✓ 1 ½ pounds green beans
- ✓ 4 garlic cloves, minced
- ✓ 1/2 tsp mustard seeds
- ✓ 1/2 tsp fennel seeds
- ✓ 1 tsp dried dill weed
- ✓ 2 tomatoes, pureed
- ✓ 1 cup cream of celery soup
- ✓ 1 tsp Italian herb mix
- ✓ 1 tsp cayenne pepper
- ✓ Salt and freshly ground black pepper

Directions:

- ❖ Heat the olive oil in a saucepan over medium flame. Once hot, fry the peppers and green beans for about 5 minutes, stirring periodically to promote even cooking.
- ❖ Add in the garlic, mustard seeds, fennel seeds and dill and continue sautéing an additional 1 minute or until fragrant.
- ❖ Add in the pureed tomatoes, cream of celery soup, Italian herb mix, cayenne pepper, salt and black pepper. Continue to simmer, covered, for about 9 minutes or until the green beans are tender.
- ❖ Taste, adjust the seasonings and serve warm. Enjoy

52) ROASTED GARDEN VEGETABLES

Preparation Time: 45 minutes

Servings: 4

Ingredients:

- ✓ 1 pound butternut squash, peeled and cut into 1-inch pieces
- ✓ 4 sweet potatoes, peeled and cut into 1-inch pieces
- ✓ 1/2 cup carrots, peeled and cut into 1-inch pieces
- ✓ 2 medium onions, cut into wedges
- ✓ 4 tbsp olive oil
- ✓ 1 tsp granulated garlic
- ✓ 1 tsp paprika
- ✓ 1 tsp dried rosemary
- ✓ 1 tsp mustard seeds
- ✓ Kosher salt and freshly ground black pepper, to taste

Directions:

- ❖ Start by preheating your oven to 420 degrees F.
- ❖ Toss the vegetables with the olive oil and spices. Arrange them on a parchment-lined roasting pan.
- ❖ Roast for about 25 minutes. Stir the vegetables and continue to cook for 20 minutes more.
- ❖ Enjoy

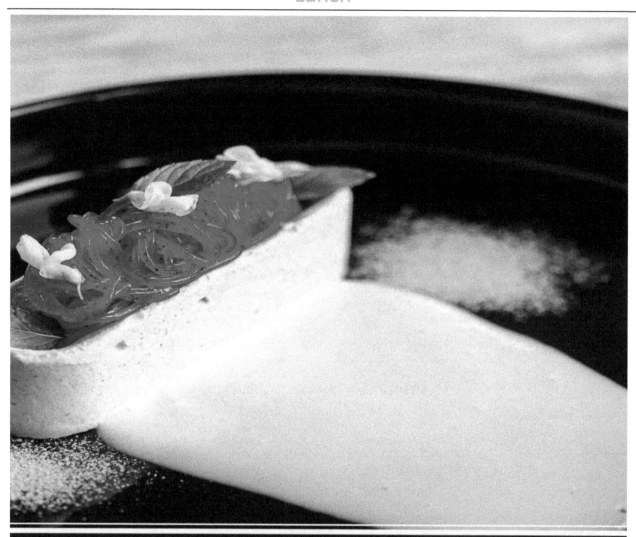

LUNCH

53) FOCACCIA WITH MIXED MUSHROOMS

Preparation Time: 35 minutes

Servings: 4

Ingredients:

- ✓ 2 tbsp flax seed powder
- ✓ ½ cup tofu mayonnaise
- ✓ ¾ cup almond flour
- ✓ 1 tbsp psyllium husk powder
- ✓ 1 tsp baking powder
- ✓ 2 oz mixed mushrooms, sliced
- ✓ 1 tbsp plant-based basil pesto
- ✓ 2 tbsp olive oil
- ✓ Salt and black pepper to taste
- ✓ ½ cup coconut cream
- ✓ ¾ cup grated plant-based Parmesan

Directions:

- ❖ Preheat oven to 350 F.
- ❖ Combine flax seed powder with 6 tbsp water and allow sitting to thicken for 5 minutes. Whisk in tofu mayonnaise, almond flour, psyllium husk powder, baking powder, and salt. Allow sitting for 5 minutes. Pour the batter into a baking sheet and spread out with a spatula. Bake for 10 minutes.
- ❖ In a bowl, mix mushrooms with pesto, olive oil, salt, and black pepper. Remove the crust from the oven and spread the coconut cream on top. Add the mushroom mixture and plant-based Parmesan cheese. Bake the pizza further until the cheese has melted, 5-10 minutes. Slice and serve with salad

54) SEITAN CAKES WITH BROCCOLI MASH

Preparation Time: 30 minutes

Servings: 4

Ingredients:

- ✓ 1 tbsp flax seed powder
- ✓ 1 ½ lb crumbled seitan
- ✓ ½ white onion
- ✓ 2 oz olive oil
- ✓ 1 lb broccoli
- ✓ 5 oz cold plant butter
- ✓ 2 oz grated plant-based Parmesan
- ✓ 4 oz plant butter, room temperature
- ✓ 2 tbsp lemon juice

Directions:

- ❖ Preheat oven to 220 F. In a bowl, mix the flax seed powder with 3 tbsp water and allow sitting to thicken for 5 minutes. When the vegan "flax egg" is ready, add in crumbled seitan, white onion, salt, and pepper. Mix and mold out 6-8 cakes out of the mixture. Melt plant butter in a skillet and fry the patties on both sides until golden brown. Remove onto a wire rack to cool slightly.
- ❖ Pour salted water into a pot, bring to a boil, and add in broccoli. Cook until the broccoli is tender but not too soft. Drain and transfer to a bowl. Add in cold plant butter, plant-based Parmesan, salt, and pepper. Puree the ingredients until smooth and creamy. Set aside. Mix the soft plant butter with lemon juice, salt, and pepper in a bowl. Serve the seitan cakes with the broccoli mash and lemon butter

55) SPICY CHEESE WITH TOFU BALLS

Preparation Time: 40 minutes

Servings: 4

Ingredients:

- ✓ 1/3 cup tofu mayonnaise
- ✓ ¼ cup pickled jalapenos
- ✓ 1 tsp paprika powder
- ✓ 1 tbsp mustard powder
- ✓ 1 pinch cayenne pepper
- ✓ 4 oz grated plant-based cheddar
- ✓ 1 tbsp flax seed powder
- ✓ 2 ½ cup crumbled tofu
- ✓ 2 tbsp plant butter

Directions:

- ❖ In a bowl, mix tofu mayonnaise, jalapeños, paprika, mustard powder, cayenne powder, and plant-based cheddar cheese; set aside. In another bowl, combine flax seed powder with 3 tbsp water and allow absorbing for 5 minutes. Add the vegan "flax egg" to the cheese mixture, crumbled tofu, salt, and pepper and combine well. Form meatballs out of the mix. Melt plant butter in a skillet and fry the tofu balls until browned. Serve the tofu balls with roasted cauliflower mash

56) QUINOA AND VEGGIE BURGERS

Preparation Time: 35 minutes

Servings: 4

Ingredients:

- 1 cup quick-cooking quinoa
- 1 tbsp olive oil
- 1 shallot, chopped
- 2 tbsp chopped fresh celery
- 1 garlic clove, minced
- 1 (15 oz) can pinto beans, drained
- 2 tbsp whole-wheat flour
- ¼ cup chopped fresh basil
- 2 tbsp pure maple syrup
- 4 whole-grain hamburger buns, split
- 4 small lettuce leaves for topping
- ½ cup tofu mayonnaise for topping

Directions:

- Cook the quinoa with 2 cups of water in a medium pot until the liquid absorbs, 10 to 15 minutes. Heat the olive oil in a medium skillet over medium heat and sauté the shallot, celery, and garlic until softened and fragrant, 3 minutes.
- Transfer the quinoa and shallot mixture to a medium bowl and add the pinto beans, flour, basil, maple syrup, salt, and black pepper. Mash and mold 4 patties out of the mixture and set aside.
- Heat a grill pan to medium heat and lightly grease with cooking spray. Cook the patties on both sides until light brown, compacted, and cooked through, 10 minutes. Place the patties between the burger buns and top with the lettuce and tofu mayonnaise. Serve

57) BAKED TOFU WITH ROASTED PEPPERS

Preparation Time: 20 minutes

Servings: 4

Ingredients:

- 3 oz cashew cream cheese
- ¾ cup tofu mayonnaise
- 2 oz cucumber, diced
- 1 large tomato, chopped
- 2 tsp dried parsley
- 4 medium orange bell peppers
- 2 ½ cups cubed tofu
- 1 tbsp melted plant butter
- 1 tsp dried basil

Directions:

- Preheat the oven's broiler to 450 F and line a baking sheet with parchment paper. In a salad bowl, combine cashew cream cheese, tofu mayonnaise, cucumber, tomato, salt, pepper, and parsley. Refrigerate.
- Arrange the bell peppers and tofu on the baking sheet, drizzle with melted plant butter, and season with basil, salt, and pepper. Bake for 10-15 minutes or until the peppers have charred lightly and the tofu browned. Remove from the oven and serve with the salad

58) ZOODLE BOLOGNESE

Preparation Time: 45 minutes

Servings: 4

Ingredients:

- 3 oz olive oil
- 1 white onion, chopped
- 1 garlic clove, minced
- 3 oz carrots, chopped
- 3 cups crumbled tofu
- 2 tbsp tomato paste
- 1 ½ cups crushed tomatoes
- Salt and black pepper to taste
- 1 tbsp dried basil
- 1 tbsp vegan Worcestershire sauce
- 2 lb zucchini, spiralized
- 2 tbsp plant butter

Directions:

- Pour olive oil into a saucepan and heat over medium heat. Add in onion, garlic, and carrots and sauté for 3 minutes or until the onions are soft and the carrots caramelized. Pour in tofu, tomato paste, tomatoes, salt, pepper, basil, and Worcestershire sauce. Stir and cook for 15 minutes. Mix in some water if the mixture is too thick and simmer further for 20 minutes. Melt plant butter in a skillet and toss in the zoodles quickly, about 1 minute. Season with salt and black pepper. Divide into serving plates and spoon the Bolognese on top. Serve immediately

59) ZUCCHINI BOATS WITH VEGAN CHEESE

Preparation Time: 40 minutes

Servings: 2

Ingredients:

- 1 medium-sized zucchini
- 4 tbsp plant butter
- 2 garlic cloves, minced
- 1 ½ oz baby kale
- Salt and black pepper to taste
- 2 tbsp unsweetened tomato sauce
- 1 cup grated plant-based mozzarella
- Olive oil for drizzling

Directions:

- Preheat oven to 375 F.
- Use a knife to slice the zucchini in halves and scoop out the pulp with a spoon into a plate. Keep the flesh. Grease a baking sheet with cooking spray and place the zucchini boats on top. Put the plant butter in a skillet and melt over medium heat.
- Sauté the garlic for 1 minute. Add in kale and zucchini pulp. Cook until the kale wilts; season with salt and black pepper. Spoon tomato sauce into the boats and spread to coat the bottom evenly. Then, spoon the kale mixture into the zucchinis and sprinkle with the plant-based mozzarella cheese. Bake for 20-25 minutes. Serve immediately

60) ROASTED BUTTERNUT SQUASH WITH CHIMICHURRI

Preparation Time: 15 minutes

Servings: 4

Ingredients:

- Zest and juice of 1 lemon
- ½ medium red bell pepper, chopped
- 1 jalapeno pepper, chopped
- 1 cup olive oil
- ½ cup chopped fresh parsley
- 2 garlic cloves, minced
- 1 lb butternut squash
- 1 tbsp plant butter, melted
- 3 tbsp toasted pine nuts

Directions:

- In a bowl, add the lemon zest and juice, red bell pepper, jalapeno, olive oil, parsley, garlic, salt, and black pepper. Use an immersion blender to grind the ingredients until your desired consistency is achieved; set aside the chimichurri.
- Slice the butternut squash into rounds and remove the seeds. Drizzle with the plant butter and season with salt and black pepper. Preheat a grill pan over medium heat and cook the squash for 2 minutes on each side or until browned. Remove the squash to serving plates, scatter the pine nuts on top, and serve with the chimichurri and red cabbage salad

61) SWEET AND SPICY BRUSSEL SPROUT STIR-FRY

Preparation Time: 15 minutes

Servings: 4

Ingredients:

- 4 oz plant butter + more to taste
- 4 shallots, chopped
- 1 tbsp apple cider vinegar
- Salt and black pepper to taste
- 1 lb Brussels sprouts
- Hot chili sauce

Directions:

- Put the plant butter in a saucepan and melt over medium heat. Pour in the shallots and sauté for 2 minutes, to caramelize and slightly soften. Add the apple cider vinegar, salt, and black pepper. Stir and reduce the heat to cook the shallots further with continuous stirring, about 5 minutes. Transfer to a plate after.
- Trim the Brussel sprouts and cut in halves. Leave the small ones as wholes. Pour the Brussel sprouts into the saucepan and stir-fry with more plant butter until softened but al dente. Season with salt and black pepper, stir in the onions and hot chili sauce, and heat for a few seconds. Serve immediately

62) BLACK BEAN BURGERS WITH BBQ SAUCE

Preparation Time: 20 minutes

Servings: 4

Ingredients:

- 3 (15 oz) cans black beans, drained
- 2 tbsp whole-wheat flour
- 2 tbsp quick-cooking oats
- ¼ cup chopped fresh basil
- 2 tbsp pure barbecue sauce
- 1 garlic clove, minced
- Salt and black pepper to taste
- 4 whole-grain hamburger buns, split
- For topping:
- Red onion slices
- Tomato slices
- Fresh basil leaves
- Additional barbecue sauce

Directions:

- In a medium bowl, mash the black beans and mix in the flour, oats, basil, barbecue sauce, garlic salt, and black pepper until well combined. Mold 4 patties out of the mixture and set aside.
- Heat a grill pan to medium heat and lightly grease with cooking spray. Cook the bean patties on both sides until light brown and cooked through, 10 minutes. Place the patties between the burger buns and top with the onions, tomatoes, basil, and some barbecue sauce. Serve warm

63) CREAMY BRUSSELS SPROUTS BAKE

Preparation Time: 26 minutes

Servings: 4

Ingredients:

- 3 tbsp plant butter
- 1 cup tempeh, cut into 1-inch cubes
- 1 ½ lb halved Brussels sprouts
- 5 garlic cloves, minced
- 1 ¼ cups coconut cream
- 10 oz grated plant-based mozzarella
- ¼ cup grated plant-based Parmesan
- Salt and black pepper to taste

Directions:

- Preheat oven to 400 F.
- Melt the plant butter in a large skillet over medium heat and fry the tempeh cubes until browned on both sides, about 6 minutes. Remove onto a plate and set aside. Pour the Brussels sprouts and garlic into the skillet and sauté until fragrant.
- Mix in coconut cream and simmer for 4 minutes. Add tempeh cubes and combine well. Pour the sauté into a baking dish, sprinkle with plant-based mozzarella cheese, and plant-based Parmesan cheese. Bake for 10 minutes or until golden brown on top. Serve with tomato salad

64) BASIL PESTO SEITAN PANINI

Preparation Time: 15 minutes+ cooling time   Servings: 4

Ingredients:

- ✓ For the seitan:
- ✓ 2/3 cup basil pesto
- ✓ ½ lemon, juiced
- ✓ 1 garlic clove, minced
- ✓ 1/8 tsp salt
- ✓ 1 cup chopped seitan

- ✓ For the panini:
- ✓ 3 tbsp basil pesto
- ✓ 8 thick slices whole-wheat ciabatta
- ✓ Olive oil for brushing
- ✓ 8 slices plant-based mozzarella
- ✓ 1 yellow bell pepper, chopped
- ✓ ¼ cup grated plant Parmesan cheese

Directions:

- ❖ In a medium bowl, mix the pesto, lemon juice, garlic, and salt. Add the seitan and coat well with the marinade. Cover with plastic wrap and marinate in the refrigerator for 30 minutes.
- ❖ Preheat a large skillet over medium heat and remove the seitan from the fridge. Cook the seitan in the skillet until brown and cooked through, 2-3 minutes. Turn the heat off.
- ❖ Preheat a panini press to medium heat. In a small bowl, mix the pesto in the inner parts of two slices of bread. On the outer parts, apply some olive oil and place a slice with (the olive oil side down) in the press. Lay 2 slices of plant-based mozzarella cheese on the bread, spoon some seitan on top. Sprinkle with some bell pepper and some plant-based Parmesan cheese. Cover with another bread slice.
- ❖ Close the press and grill the bread for 1 to 2 minutes. Flip the bread, and grill further for 1 minute or until the cheese melts and golden brown on both sides. Serve warm

65) SWEET OATMEAL "GRITS"

Preparation Time: 20 minutes   Servings: 4

Ingredients:

- ✓ 1 ½ cups steel-cut oats, soaked overnight
- ✓ 1 cup almond milk
- ✓ 2 cups water
- ✓ A pinch of grated nutmeg

- ✓ A pinch of ground cloves
- ✓ A pinch of sea salt
- ✓ 4 tbsp almonds, slivered
- ✓ 6 dates, pitted and chopped
- ✓ 6 prunes, chopped

Directions:

- ❖ In a deep saucepan, bring the steel cut oats, almond milk and water to a boil.
- ❖ Add in the nutmeg, cloves and salt. Immediately turn the heat to a simmer, cover and continue to cook for about 15 minutes or until they've softened.
- ❖ Then, spoon the grits into four serving bowls; top them with the almonds, dates and prunes.
- ❖ Enjoy!

66) FREEKEH BOWL WITH DRIED FIGS

Preparation Time: 35 minutes   Servings: 2

Ingredients:

- ✓ 1/2 cup freekeh, soaked for 30 minutes, drained
- ✓ 1 1/3 cups almond milk
- ✓ 1/4 tsp sea salt

- ✓ 1/4 tsp ground cloves
- ✓ 1/4 tsp ground cinnamon
- ✓ 4 tbsp agave syrup
- ✓ 2 ounces dried figs, chopped

Directions:

- ❖ Place the freekeh, milk, sea salt, ground cloves and cinnamon in a saucepan. Bring to a boil over medium-high heat.
- ❖ Immediately turn the heat to a simmer for 30 to 35 minutes, stirring occasionally to promote even cooking.
- ❖ Stir in the agave syrup and figs. Ladle the porridge into individual bowls and serve. Enjoy

67) CORNMEAL PORRIDGE WITH MAPLE SYRUP

Preparation Time: 20 minutes   Servings: 4

Ingredients:

- ✓ 2 cups water
- ✓ 2 cups almond milk
- ✓ 1 cinnamon stick

- ✓ 1 vanilla bean
- ✓ 1 cup yellow cornmeal
- ✓ 1/2 cup maple syrup

Directions:

- ❖ In a saucepan, bring the water and almond milk to a boil. Add in the cinnamon stick and vanilla bean.
- ❖ Gradually add in the cornmeal, stirring continuously; turn the heat to a simmer. Let it simmer for about 15 minutes.
- ❖ Drizzle the maple syrup over the porridge and serve warm. Enjoy

68) MEDITERRANEAN-STYLE RICE

Preparation Time: 20 minutes

Servings: 4

Ingredients:

- ✓ 3 tbsp vegan butter, at room temperature
- ✓ 4 tbsp scallions, chopped
- ✓ 2 cloves garlic, minced
- ✓ 1 bay leaf
- ✓ 1 thyme sprig, chopped
- ✓ 1 rosemary sprig, chopped
- ✓ 1 ½ cups white rice
- ✓ 2 cups vegetable broth
- ✓ 1 large tomato, pureed
- ✓ Sea salt and ground black pepper, to taste
- ✓ 2 ounces Kalamata olives, pitted and sliced

Directions:

- ❖ In a saucepan, melt the vegan butter over a moderately high flame. Cook the scallions for about 2 minutes or until tender.
- ❖ Add in the garlic, bay leaf, thyme and rosemary and continue to sauté for about 1 minute or until aromatic.
- ❖ Add in the rice, broth and pureed tomato. Bring to a boil; immediately turn the heat to a gentle simmer.
- ❖ Cook for about 15 minutes or until all the liquid has absorbed. Fluff the rice with a fork, season with salt and pepper and garnish with olives; serve immediately. Enjoy

69) BULGUR PANCAKES WITH A TWIST

Preparation Time: 50 minutes

Servings: 4

Ingredients:

- ✓ 1/2 cup bulgur wheat flour
- ✓ 1/2 cup almond flour
- ✓ 1 tsp baking soda
- ✓ 1/2 tsp fine sea salt
- ✓ 1 cup full-fat coconut milk
- ✓ 1/2 tsp ground cinnamon
- ✓ 1/4 tsp ground cloves
- ✓ 4 tbsp coconut oil
- ✓ 1/2 cup maple syrup
- ✓ 1 large-sized banana, sliced

Directions:

- ❖ In a mixing bowl, thoroughly combine the flour, baking soda, salt, coconut milk, cinnamon and ground cloves; let it stand for 30 minutes to soak well.
- ❖ Heat a small amount of the coconut oil in a frying pan.
- ❖ Fry the pancakes until the surface is golden brown. Garnish with maple syrup and banana. Enjoy

70) CHOCOLATE RYE PORRIDGE

Preparation Time: 10 minutes

Servings: 4

Ingredients:

- ✓ 2 cups rye flakes
- ✓ 2 ½ cups almond milk
- ✓ 2 ounces dried prunes, chopped
- ✓ 2 ounces dark chocolate chunks

Directions:

- ❖ Add the rye flakes and almond milk to a deep saucepan; bring to a boil over medium-high. Turn the heat to a simmer and let it cook for 5 to 6 minutes.
- ❖ Remove from the heat. Fold in the chopped prunes and chocolate chunks, gently stir to combine.
- ❖ Ladle into serving bowls and serve warm.
- ❖ Enjoy

71) AUTHENTIC AFRICAN MIELIE-MEAL

Preparation Time: 15 minutes

Servings: 4

Ingredients:

- ✓ 3 cups water
- ✓ 1 cup coconut milk
- ✓ 1 cup maize meal
- ✓ 1/3 tsp kosher salt
- ✓ 1/4 tsp grated nutmeg
- ✓ 1/4 tsp ground cloves
- ✓ 4 tbsp maple syrup

Directions:

- ❖ In a saucepan, bring the water and milk to a boil; then, gradually add in the maize meal and turn the heat to a simmer.
- ❖ Add in the salt, nutmeg and cloves. Let it cook for 10 minutes.
- ❖ Add in the maple syrup and gently stir to combine. Enjoy

72) TEFF PORRIDGE WITH DRIED FIGS

Preparation Time: 25 minutes

Servings: 4

Ingredients:

- 1 cup whole-grain teff
- 1 cup water
- 2 cups coconut milk
- 2 tbsp coconut oil
- 1/2 tsp ground cardamom
- 1/4 tsp ground cinnamon
- 4 tbsp agave syrup
- 7-8 dried figs, chopped

Directions:

- Bring the whole-grain teff, water and coconut milk to a boil.
- Turn the heat to a simmer and add in the coconut oil, cardamom and cinnamon.
- Let it cook for 20 minutes or until the grain has softened and the porridge has thickened. Stir in the agave syrup and stir to combine well.
- Top each serving bowl with chopped figs and serve warm. Enjoy

73) DECADENT BREAD PUDDING WITH APRICOTS

Preparation Time: 1 hour

Servings: 4

Ingredients:

- 4 cups day-old ciabatta bread, cubed
- 4 tbsp coconut oil, melted
- 2 cups coconut milk
- 1/2 cup coconut sugar
- 4 tbsp applesauce
- 1/4 tsp ground cloves
- 1/2 tsp ground cinnamon
- 1 tsp vanilla extract
- 1/3 cup dried apricots, diced

Directions:

- Start by preheating your oven to 360 degrees F. Lightly oil a casserole dish with a nonstick cooking spray.
- Place the cubed bread in the prepared casserole dish.
- In a mixing bowl, thoroughly combine the coconut oil, milk, coconut sugar, applesauce, ground cloves, ground cinnamon and vanilla. Pour the custard evenly over the bread cubes; fold in the apricots.
- Press with a wide spatula and let it soak for about 15 minutes.
- Bake in the preheated oven for about 45 minutes or until the top is golden and set. Enjoy

74) CHIPOTLE CILANTRO RICE

Preparation Time: 25 minutes

Servings: 4

Ingredients:

- 4 tbsp olive oil
- 1 chipotle pepper, seeded and chopped
- 1 cup jasmine rice
- 1 ½ cups vegetable broth
- 1/4 cup fresh cilantro, chopped
- Sea salt and cayenne pepper, to taste

Directions:

- In a saucepan, heat the olive oil over a moderately high flame. Add in the pepper and rice and cook for about 3 minutes or until aromatic.
- Pour the vegetable broth into the saucepan and bring to a boil; immediately turn the heat to a gentle simmer.
- Cook for about 18 minutes or until all the liquid has absorbed. Fluff the rice with a fork, add in the cilantro, salt and cayenne pepper; stir to combine well. Enjoy

75) OAT PORRIDGE WITH ALMONDS

Preparation Time: 20 minutes

Servings: 2

Ingredients:

- 1 cup water
- 2 cups almond milk, divided
- 1 cup rolled oats
- 2 tbsp coconut sugar
- 1/2 vanilla essence
- 1/4 tsp cardamom
- 1/2 cup almonds, chopped
- 1 banana, sliced

Directions:

- In a deep saucepan, bring the water and milk to a rapid boil. Add in the oats, cover the saucepan and turn the heat to medium.
- Add in the coconut sugar, vanilla and cardamom. Continue to cook for about 12 minutes, stirring periodically.
- Spoon the mixture into serving bowls; top with almonds and banana. Enjoy

76) AROMATIC MILLET BOWL

Preparation Time: 20 minutes

Servings: 3

Ingredients:

- 1 cup water
- 1 ½ cups coconut milk
- 1 cup millet, rinsed and drained
- 1/4 tsp crystallized ginger
- 1/4 tsp ground cinnamon
- A pinch of grated nutmeg
- A pinch of Himalayan salt
- 2 tbsp maple syrup

Directions:

- Place the water, milk, millet, crystallized ginger cinnamon, nutmeg and salt in a saucepan; bring to a boil.
- Turn the heat to a simmer and let it cook for about 20 minutes; fluff the millet with a fork and spoon into individual bowls.
- Serve with maple syrup. Enjoy

77) HARISSA BULGUR BOWL

Preparation Time: 25 minutes

Servings: 4

Ingredients:

- 1 cup bulgur wheat
- 1 ½ cups vegetable broth
- 2 cups sweet corn kernels, thawed
- 1 cup canned kidney beans, drained
- 1 red onion, thinly sliced
- 1 garlic clove, minced
- Sea salt and ground black pepper, to taste
- 1/4 cup harissa paste
- 1 tbsp lemon juice
- 1 tbsp white vinegar
- 1/4 cup extra-virgin olive oil
- 1/4 cup fresh parsley leaves, roughly chopped

Directions:

- In a deep saucepan, bring the bulgur wheat and vegetable broth to a simmer; let it cook, covered, for 12 to 13 minutes.
- Let it stand for 5 to 10 minutes and fluff your bulgur with a fork.
- Add the remaining ingredients to the cooked bulgur wheat; serve warm or at room temperature. Enjoy

78) COCONUT QUINOA PUDDING

Preparation Time: 20 minutes

Servings: 3

Ingredients:

- 1 cup water
- 1 cup coconut milk
- 1 cup quinoa
- A pinch of kosher salt
- A pinch of ground allspice
- 1/2 tsp cinnamon
- 1/2 tsp vanilla extract
- 4 tbsp agave syrup
- 1/2 cup coconut flakes

Directions:

- Place the water, coconut milk, quinoa, salt, ground allspice, cinnamon and vanilla extract in a saucepan.
- Bring it to a boil over medium-high heat. Turn the heat to a simmer and let it cook for about 20 minutes; fluff with a fork and add in the agave syrup.
- Divide between three serving bowls and garnish with coconut flakes. Enjoy

79) CREMINI MUSHROOM RISOTTO

Preparation Time: 20 minutes

Servings: 3

Ingredients:

- 3 tbsp vegan butter
- 1 tsp garlic, minced
- 1 tsp thyme
- 1 pound Cremini mushrooms, sliced
- 1 ½ cups white rice
- 2 ½ cups vegetable broth
- 1/4 cup dry sherry wine
- Kosher salt and ground black pepper, to taste
- 3 tbsp fresh scallions, thinly sliced

Directions:

- In a saucepan, melt the vegan butter over a moderately high flame. Cook the garlic and thyme for about 1 minute or until aromatic.
- Add in the mushrooms and continue to sauté until they release the liquid or about 3 minutes.
- Add in the rice, vegetable broth and sherry wine. Bring to a boil; immediately turn the heat to a gentle simmer.
- Cook for about 15 minutes or until all the liquid has absorbed. Fluff the rice with a fork, season with salt and pepper and garnish with fresh scallions. Enjoy

Dinner

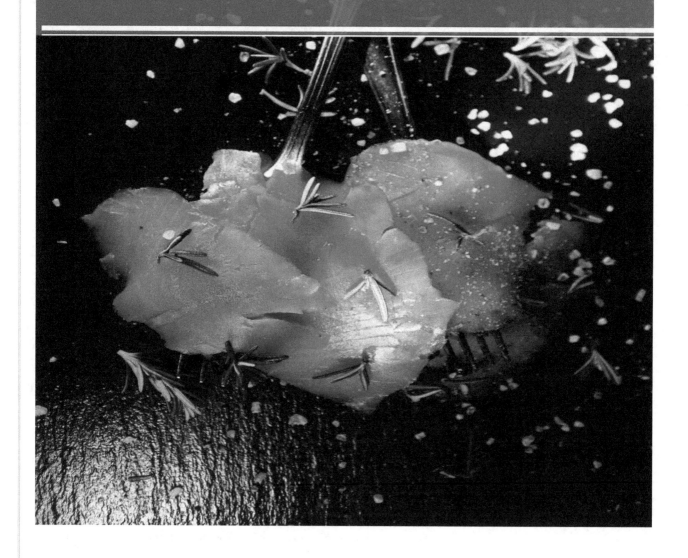

80) QUINOA AND CHICKPEA POT

Preparation Time: 15 minutes

Servings: 2

Ingredients:

- ✓ 2 tsp olive oil
- ✓ 1 cup cooked quinoa
- ✓ 1 (15-oz) can chickpeas

- ✓ 1 bunch arugula chopped
- ✓ 1 tbsp soy
- ✓ Sea salt and black pepper to taste

Directions:

- ❖ Heat the oil in a skillet over medium heat. Stir in quinoa, chickpeas, and arugula and cook for 3-5 minutes until the arugula wilts. Pour in soy sauce, salt, and pepper. Toss to coat. Serve immediately

81) BUCKWHEAT PILAF WITH PINE NUTS

Preparation Time: 25 minutes

Servings: 4

Ingredients:

- ✓ 1 cup buckwheat groats
- ✓ 2 cups vegetable stock
- ✓ ¼ cup pine nuts

- ✓ 2 tbsp olive oil
- ✓ ½ onion, chopped
- ✓ ⅓ cup chopped fresh parsley

Directions:

- ❖ Put the groats and vegetable stock in a pot. Bring to a boil, then lower the heat and simmer for 15 minutes. Heat a skillet over medium heat. Place in the pine nuts and toast for 2-3 minutes, shaking often. Heat the oil in the same skillet and sauté the onion for 3 minutes until translucent.
- ❖ Once the groats are ready, fluff them using a fork. Mix in pine nuts, onion, and parsley. Sprinkle with salt and pepper. Serve

82)

83) ITALIAN HOLIDAY STUFFING

Preparation Time: 25 minutes

Servings: 4

Ingredients:

- ✓ ¼ cup plant butter
- ✓ 1 onion, chopped
- ✓ 2 celery stalks, sliced
- ✓ 1 cup button mushrooms, sliced
- ✓ 3 garlic cloves, minced

- ✓ ½ cup vegetable broth
- ✓ ½ cup raisins
- ✓ ½ cup chopped walnuts
- ✓ 2 cups cooked quinoa
- ✓ 1 tsp Italian seasoning
- ✓ Sea salt to taste
- ✓ Chopped fresh parsley

Directions:

- ❖ In a skillet over medium heat, melt the butter. Sauté the onion, garlic, celery, and mushrooms for 5 minutes until tender, stirring occasionally. Pour in broth, raisins, and walnuts. Bring to a boil, then lower the heat and simmer for 5 minutes. Stir in quinoa, Italian seasoning, and salt. Cook for another 4 minutes. Serve garnished with parsley

84) PRESSURE COOKER GREEN LENTILS

Preparation Time: 30 minutes

Servings: 6

Ingredients:

- ✓ 3 tbsp coconut oil
- ✓ 2 tbsp curry powder
- ✓ 1 tsp ground ginger
- ✓ 1 onion, chopped

- ✓ 2 garlic cloves, sliced
- ✓ 1 cup dried green lentils
- ✓ 3 cups water
- ✓ Salt and black pepper to taste

Directions:

- ❖ Set your IP to Sauté. Add in coconut oil, curry powder, ginger, onion, and garlic. Cook for 3 minutes. Stir in green lentils. Pour in water. Lock the lid and set the time to 10 minutes on High. Once ready, perform a natural pressure release for 10 minutes. Unlock the lid and season with salt and pepper. Serve

85) CHERRY AND PISTACHIO BULGUR

Preparation Time: 45 minutes

Servings: 4

Ingredients:

- ✓ 1 tbsp plant butter
- ✓ 1 white onion, chopped
- ✓ 1 carrot, chopped
- ✓ 1 celery stalk, chopped
- ✓ 1 cup chopped mushrooms
- ✓ 1 ½ cups bulgur
- ✓ 4 cups vegetable broth
- ✓ 1 cup chopped dried cherries, soaked
- ✓ ½ cup chopped pistachios

Directions:

- ❖ Preheat oven to 375 F.
- ❖ Melt butter in a skillet over medium heat. Sauté the onion, carrot, and celery for 5 minutes until tender. Add in mushrooms and cook for 3 more minutes. Pour in bulgur and broth. Transfer to a casserole and bake covered for 30 minutes. Once ready, uncover and stir in cherries. Top with pistachios to serve

86) MUSHROOM FRIED RICE

Preparation Time: 25 minutes

Servings: 6

Ingredients:

- ✓ 2 tbsp sesame oil
- ✓ 1 onion, chopped
- ✓ 1 carrot, chopped
- ✓ 1 cup okra, chopped
- ✓ 1 cup sliced shiitake mushrooms
- ✓ 2 garlic cloves, minced
- ✓ ¼ cup soy sauce
- ✓ 1 cups cooked brown rice
- ✓ 2 green onions, chopped

Directions:

- ❖ Heat the oil in a skillet over medium heat. Place in onion and carrot and cook for 3 minutes. Add in okra and mushrooms, cook for 5-7 minutes. Stir in garlic and cook for 30 seconds. Put in soy sauce and rice. Cook until hot. Add in green onions and stir. Serve warm

87) BEAN AND BROWN RICE WITH ARTICHOKES

Preparation Time: 35 minutes

Servings: 4

Ingredients:

- ✓ 2 tbsp olive oil
- ✓ 3 garlic cloves, minced
- ✓ 1 cup artichokes hearts, chopped
- ✓ 1 tsp dried basil
- ✓ 1 ½ cups cooked navy beans
- ✓ 1 ½ cups long-grain brown rice
- ✓ 3 cups vegetable broth
- ✓ Salt and black pepper to taste
- ✓ 2 ripe grape tomatoes, quartered
- ✓ 2 tbsp minced fresh parsley

Directions:

- ❖ Heat the oil in a pot over medium heat. Sauté the garlic for 1 minute. Stir in artichokes, basil, navy beans, rice, and broth. Sprinkle with salt and pepper. Lower the heat and simmer for 20-25 minutes. Remove to a bowl and mix in tomatoes and parsley. Using a fork, fluff the rice and serve right away

88) PRESSURE COOKER CELERY AND SPINACH CHICKPEAS

Preparation Time: 50 minutes

Servings: 5

Ingredients:

- ✓ 1 cup chickpeas, soaked overnight
- ✓ 1 onion, chopped
- ✓ 2 garlic cloves, minced
- ✓ 1 celery stalk, chopped
- ✓ 2 tbsp olive oil
- ✓ 3 tsp ground cinnamon
- ✓ ½ tsp ground nutmeg
- ✓ 1 tbsp coconut oil
- ✓ 1 cup spinach, chopped

Directions:

- ❖ Place chickpeas in your IP with the onion, garlic, celery, olive oil, 2 cups water, cinnamon, and nutmeg.
- ❖ Lock the lid in place; set the time to 30 minutes on High. Once ready, perform a natural pressure release for 10 minutes. Unlock the lid and drain the excess water. Put back the chickpeas and stir in coconut oil and spinach. Set the pot to Sauté and cook for another 5 minutes

89) VEGGIE PAELLA WITH LENTILS

Preparation Time: 50 minutes

Servings: 4

Ingredients:

- 2 tbsp olive oil
- 1 onion, chopped
- 1 green bell pepper, chopped
- 2 garlic cloves, minced
- 1 (14.5-oz) can diced tomatoes
- 1 tbsp capers
- ¼ tsp crushed red pepper
- 1 ½ cups long-grain brown rice
- 3 cups vegetable broth
- 1 ½ cups cooked lentils, drained
- ¼ cup sliced pitted black olives
- 2 tbsp minced fresh parsley

Directions:

- Heat oil in a pot over medium heat and sauté onion, bell pepper, and garlic for 5 minutes. Stir in tomatoes, capers, red pepper, and salt. Cook for 5 minutes. Pour in the rice and broth. Bring to a boil, then lower the heat. Simmer for 20 minutes. Turn the heat off and mix in lentils. Serve garnished with olives and parsley

90) CURRY BEAN WITH ARTICHOKES

Preparation Time: 25 minutes

Servings: 4

Ingredients:

- 1 (14.5-oz) can artichoke hearts, drained and quartered
- 1 tsp olive oil
- 1 small onion, diced
- 2 garlic cloves, minced
- 1 (14.5-oz) can cannellini beans
- 2 tsp curry powder
- ½ tsp ground coriander
- 1 (5.4-oz) can coconut milk
- Salt and black pepper to taste

Directions:

- Heat the oil in a skillet over medium heat. Sauté the onion and garlic for 3 minutes until translucent. Stir in beans, artichoke, curry powder, and coriander. Add in coconut milk. Bring to a boil, then lower the heat and simmer for 10 minutes. Serve

91) ENDIVE SLAW WITH OLIVES

Preparation Time: 10 minutes

Servings: 6

Ingredients:

- 1 lb curly endive, chopped
- ⅓ cup vegan mayonnaise
- ¼ cup rice vinegar
- 2 tbsp vegan yogurt
- 1 tbsp pure date sugar
- 10 black olives for garnish
- ¼ tsp freshly ground black pepper
- ¼ tsp smoked paprika
- ¼ tsp chipotle powder

Directions:

- In a bowl, mix the mayonnaise, vinegar, yogurt, sugar, salt, pepper, paprika, and chipotle powder. Gently add in the curly endive and mix with a wooden spatula to coat. Top with black olives and serve

92) PAPRIKA CAULIFLOWER TACOS

Preparation Time: 40 minutes

Servings: 6

Ingredients:

- 1 head cauliflower, cut into pieces
- 2 tbsp olive oil
- 2 tbsp whole-wheat flour
- 2 tbsp nutritional yeast
- 2 tsp paprika
- 1 tsp cayenne pepper
- Salt to taste
- 1 cups shredded watercress
- 2 cups cherry tomatoes, halved
- 2 carrots, grated
- ½ cup mango salsa
- ½ cup guacamole
- 8 small corn tortillas, warm
- 1 lime, cut into wedges

Directions:

- Preheat oven to 350 F.
- Brush the cauliflower with oil in a bowl. In another bowl, mix the flour, yeast, paprika, cayenne pepper, and salt. Pour into the cauliflower bowl and toss to coat. Spread the cauliflower on a greased baking sheet. Bake for 20-30 minutes.
- In a bowl, combine the watercress, cherry tomatoes, carrots, mango salsa, and guacamole. Once the cauliflower is ready, divide it between the tortillas, add the mango mixture, roll up and serve with lime wedges on the side

93) SIMPLE PESTO MILLET

Preparation Time: 50 minutes

Servings: 4

✓ ½ cup vegan basil pesto

Ingredients:

✓ 1 cup millet
✓ 2 ½ cups vegetable broth

Directions:

❖ Place the millet and broth in a pot. Bring to a boil, then lower the heat and simmer for 25 minutes. Let cool for 5 minutes and fluff the millet. Mix in the pesto and serve

94) PEPPERED PINTO BEANS

Preparation Time: 30 minutes

Servings: 6

✓ 2 carrots, chopped
✓ 2 garlic cloves, minced
✓ 3 (15-oz) cans pinto beans
✓ 18-ounce bottle barbecue sauce
✓ ½ tsp chipotle powder

Ingredients:

✓ 1 serrano pepper, cut into strips
✓ 1 red bell pepper, cut into strips
✓ 1 green bell pepper, cut into strips
✓ 1 onion, chopped

Directions:

❖ In a blender, place the serrano and bell peppers, onion, carrot, and garlic. Pulse until well mixed.
❖ Place the mixture in a pot with the beans, BBQ sauce, and chipotle powder. Cook for 15 minutes. Season with salt and pepper. Serve warm

95) BLACK-EYED PEAS WITH SUN-DRIED TOMATOES

Preparation Time: 35 minutes

Servings: 4

✓ 1 ½ tsp ground cumin
✓ 1 ½ tsp onion powder
✓ 1 tsp dried oregano
✓ ¾ tsp garlic powder
✓ ½ tsp smoked paprika

Ingredients:

✓ 1 cup black-eyed peas, soaked overnight
✓ ¼ cup sun-dried tomatoes, chopped
✓ 2 tbsp olive oil
✓ 2 tsp ground chipotle pepper

Directions:

❖ Place the black-eyed peas in a pot and add 2 cups of water, olive oil, chipotle pepper, cumin, onion powder, oregano, garlic powder, salt, and paprika. Cook for 20 minutes over medium heat. Mix in sun-dried tomatoes, let sit for a few minutes and serve

96) VEGETARIAN QUINOA CURRY

Preparation Time: 35 minutes

Servings: 4

✓ 1 cup canned diced tomatoes
✓ 4 cups chopped spinach
✓ ½ cup non-dairy milk
✓ 2 tbsp soy sauce
✓ Salt to taste

Ingredients:

✓ 4 tsp olive oil
✓ 1 onion, chopped
✓ 2 tbsp curry powder
✓ 1 ½ cups quinoa

Directions:

❖ Heat the oil in a pot over medium heat. Sauté the onion and ginger for 3 minutes until tender. Pour in curry powder, quinoa, and 3 cups of water. Bring to a boil, then lower the heat and simmer for 15-20 minutes. Mix in tomatoes, spinach, milk, soy sauce, and salt. Simmer for an additional 3 minutes

97) ALFREDO RICE WITH GREEN BEANS

Preparation Time: 25 minutes

Servings: 3

✓ 2 cups brown rice

Ingredients:

✓ 1 cup Alfredo arugula vegan pesto
✓ 1 cup frozen green beans, thawed

Directions:

❖ Cook the rice in salted water in a pot over medium heat for 20 minutes. Drain and let it cool completely. Place the Alfredo sauce and beans in a skillet. Cook over low heat for 3-5 minutes. Stir in the rice to coat. Serve immediately

98) KOREAN-STYLE MILLET

Preparation Time: 30 minutes

Servings: 4

Ingredients:

- ✓ 1 cup dried millet, drained
- ✓ 1 tsp gochugaru flakes
- ✓ Salt and black pepper to taste

Directions:

- ❖ Place the millet and gochugaru flakes in a pot. Cover with enough water and bring to a boil. Lower the heat and simmer for 20 minutes. Drain and let cool. Transfer to a serving bowl and season with salt and pepper. Serve

99) LEMONY CHICKPEAS WITH KALE

Preparation Time: 20 minutes

Servings: 4

Ingredients:

- ✓ 4 tbsp olive oil
- ✓ 1 (15-oz) can chickpeas
- ✓ 1 onion, chopped
- ✓ 2 garlic cloves, minced
- ✓ 1 tbsp Italian seasoning
- ✓ 2 cups kale, chopped
- ✓ Sea salt and black pepper to taste
- ✓ Juice and zest of 1 lemon

Directions:

- ❖ Heat the oil in a skillet over medium heat. Place in chickpeas and cook for 5 minutes. Add in onion, garlic, Italian seasoning, and kale and cook for 5 minutes until the kale wilts. Stir in salt, lemon juice, lemon zest, and pepper. Serve warm

100) DINNER RICE AND LENTILS

Preparation Time: 25 minutes

Servings: 4

Ingredients:

- ✓ 2 tbsp olive oil
- ✓ 4 scallions, chopped
- ✓ 1 carrot, diced
- ✓ 1 celery stalk, chopped
- ✓ 2 (15-oz) cans lentils, drained
- ✓ 1 (15-oz) can diced tomatoes
- ✓ 1 tbsp dried rosemary
- ✓ 1 tsp ground coriander
- ✓ 1 tbsp garlic powder
- ✓ 2 cups cooked brown rice
- ✓ Sea salt and black pepper to taste

Directions:

- ❖ Heat the oil in a pot over medium heat. Place in scallions, carrot, and celery and cook for 5 minutes until tender. Stir in lentils, tomatoes, rosemary, coriander, and garlic powder. Lower the heat and simmer for 5-7 minutes. Mix in rice, salt, and pepper and cook another 2-3 minutes. Serve

101) SESAME KALE SLAW

Preparation Time: 15 minutes

Servings: 4

Ingredients:

- ✓ ¼ cup tahini
- ✓ 2 tbsp white miso paste
- ✓ 1 tbsp rice vinegar
- ✓ 1 tbsp toasted sesame oil
- ✓ 2 tsp soy sauce
- ✓ 1 (12-oz) bag kale slaw
- ✓ 2 scallions, minced
- ✓ ¼ cup toasted sesame seeds

Directions:

- ❖ In a bowl, combine the tahini, miso, vinegar, oil, and soy sauce. Stir in kale slaw, scallions, and sesame seeds. Let sit for 20 minutes. Serve immediately

102) SPICY STEAMED BROCCOLI

Preparation Time: 15 minutes

Servings: 6

Ingredients:

- ✓ 1 large head broccoli, into florets
- ✓ Salt to taste
- ✓ **1 tsp red pepper flakes**

Directions:

- ❖ Boil 1 cup water in a pot over medium heat. Place in a steamer basket and put in the florets. Steam covered for 5-7 minutes. In a bowl, toss the broccoli with red pepper flakes and salt. Serve

103) GARLIC ROASTED CARROTS

Preparation Time: 35 minutes

Servings: 4

Ingredients:

- ✓ 2 lb carrots, chopped into ¾ inch cubes
- ✓ 2 tsp olive oil
- ✓ ½ tsp chili powder
- ✓ ½ tsp smoked paprika
- ✓ ½ tsp dried oregano
- ✓ ½ tsp dried thyme
- ✓ ½ tsp garlic powder
- ✓ Salt to taste

Directions:

- ❖ Preheat oven to 400 F. Line with parchment paper a baking sheet. Rinse the carrots and pat dry. Chop into ¾ inch cubes. Place in a bowl and toss with olive oil.
- ❖ In a bowl, mix chili powder, paprika, oregano, thyme, olive oil, salt, and garlic powder. Pour over the carrots and toss to coat. Transfer to a greased baking sheet and bake for 30 minutes, turn once by half

104) EGGPLANT AND HUMMUS PIZZA

Preparation Time: 25 minutes

Servings: 2

Ingredients:

- ✓ ½ eggplant, sliced
- ✓ ½ red onion, sliced
- ✓ 1 cup cherry tomatoes, halved
- ✓ 3 tbsp chopped black olives
- ✓ Salt to taste
- ✓ Drizzle olive oil
- ✓ 2 prebaked pizza crusts
- ✓ ½ cup hummus
- ✓ 2 tbsp oregano

Directions:

- ❖ Preheat oven to 390 F,
- ❖ In a bowl, combine the eggplant, onion, tomatoes, olives, and salt. Toss to coat. Sprinkle with some olive oil. Arrange the crusts on a baking sheet and spread the hummus on each pizza. Top with the eggplant mixture. Bake for 20-30 minutes. Serve warm

105) MISO GREEN CABBAGE

Preparation Time: 50 minutes

Servings: 4

Ingredients:

- ✓ 1 lb green cabbage, halved
- ✓ 2 tsp olive
- ✓ 3 tsp miso paste
- ✓ 1 tsp dried oregano
- ✓ ½ tsp dried rosemary
- ✓ 1 tbsp balsamic vinegar

Directions:

- ❖ Preheat oven to 390 F. Line with parchment paper a baking sheet.
- ❖ Put the green cabbage in a bowl. Coat with olive oil, miso, oregano, rosemary, salt, and pepper. Remove to the baking sheet and bake for 35-40 minutes, shaking every 5 minutes until tender. Remove from the oven to a plate. Drizzle with balsamic vinegar and serve

106) STEAMED BROCCOLI WITH HAZELNUTS

Preparation Time: 20 minutes

Servings: 4

Ingredients:

- ✓ 1 lb broccoli, cut into florets
- ✓ 2 tbsp olive oil
- ✓ 3 garlic cloves, minced
- ✓ 1 cup sliced white mushrooms
- ✓ ¼ cup dry white wine
- ✓ 2 tbsp minced fresh parsley
- ✓ Salt and black pepper to taste
- ✓ ½ cup slivered toasted hazelnuts

Directions:

- ❖ Steam the broccoli for 8 minutes or until tender. Remove and set aside.
- ❖ Heat 1 tbsp of oil in a skillet over medium heat. Add in garlic and mushrooms and sauté for 5 minutes until tender. Pour in the wine and cook for 1 minute. Stir in broccoli, parsley, salt, and pepper. Cook for 3 minutes, until the liquid has reduced. Remove to a bowl and add in the remaining oil and hazelnuts and toss to coat. Serve warm

107) CILANTRO OKRA

Preparation Time: 10 minutes

Servings: 4

Ingredients:

- ✓ 2 tbsp olive oil
- ✓ 4 cups okra, halved
- ✓ Sea salt and black pepper to taste
- ✓ 3 tbsp chopped fresh cilantro

Directions:

- ❖ Heat the oil in a skillet over medium heat. Place in the okra, cook for 5 minutes. Turn the heat off and mix in salt, pepper, and cilantro. Serve immediately

108) CITRUS ASPARAGUS

Preparation Time: 15 minutes

Servings: 4

Ingredients:

- ✓ 1 onion, minced
- ✓ 2 tsp lemon zest
- ✓ 1/3 cup fresh lemon juice
- ✓ 1 tbsp olive oil
- ✓ Salt and black pepper to taste
- ✓ 1 lb asparagus, trimmed

Directions:

- ❖ Combine the onion, lemon zest, lemon juice, and oil in a bowl. Sprinkle with salt and pepper. Let sit for 5-10 minutes.
- ❖ Insert a steamer basket and 1 cup of water in a pot over medium heat. Place the asparagus on the basket and steam for 4-5 minutes until tender but crispy. Leave to cool for 10 minutes, then arrange on a plate. Serve drizzled with the dressing

109) JAPANESE-STYLE TOFU WITH HARICOTS VERT

Preparation Time: 25 minutes

Servings: 4

Ingredients:

- ✓ 1 cup haricots vert
- ✓ 1 tbsp grapeseed oil
- ✓ 1 onion, minced
- ✓ 5 shiitake mushroom caps, sliced
- ✓ 1 tsp grated fresh ginger
- ✓ 3 green onions, minced
- ✓ 8 oz firm tofu, crumbled
- ✓ 2 tbsp soy sauce
- ✓ 3 cups hot cooked rice
- ✓ 1 tbsp toasted sesame oil
- ✓ 1 tbsp toasted sesame seeds

Directions:

- ❖ Place the haricots in boiled salted water and cook for 10 minutes until tender. Drain and set aside.
- ❖ Heat the oil in a skillet over medium heat. Place in onion and cook for 3 minutes until translucent. Add in mushrooms, ginger, green onions, tofu, and soy sauce. Cook for 10 minutes. Share into 4 bowls and top with haricot and tofu mixture. Sprinkle with sesame oil. Serve garnished with sesame seeds

110) RAISIN AND ORZO STUFFED TOMATOES

Preparation Time: 40 minutes

Servings: 4

Ingredients:

- ✓ 2 cups cooked orzo
- ✓ Salt and black pepper to taste
- ✓ 3 green onions, minced
- ✓ 1/3 cup golden raisins
- ✓ 1 tsp orange zest
- ✓ 4 large ripe tomatoes
- ✓ 1/3 cup toasted pine nuts
- ✓ ¼ cup minced fresh parsley
- ✓ 2 tsp olive oil

Directions:

- ❖ Preheat oven to 380 F.
- ❖ Mix the orzo, green onions, raisins, and orange zest in a bowl. Set aside. Slice the top of the tomato by ½-inch and take out the pulp. Cut the pulp and place it in a bowl. Stir in orzo mixture, pine nuts, parsley, salt, and pepper.
- ❖ Spoon the mixture into the tomatoes and arrange on a greased baking tray. Sprinkle with oil and cover with foil. Bake for 15 minutes. Uncover and bake for another 5 minutes until golden

111) ROSEMARY BAKED POTATOES WITH CHERRY TOMATOES

Preparation Time: 65 minutes

Servings: 5

Ingredients:

- ✓ 5 russet potatoes, sliced
- ✓ ½ cup cherry tomatoes, halved
- ✓ 2 tbsp rosemary
- ✓ 2 tbsp olive oil
- ✓ Salt and black pepper to taste

Directions:

- ❖ Preheat oven to 390 F. Make several incisions with a fork in each potato. Rub each potato and cherry tomatoes with olive oil and sprinkle with salt, rosemary, and pepper. Arrange on a baking dish and bake for 50-60 minutes. Once ready, transfer to a rack and allow to completely cool before serving

SNACKS

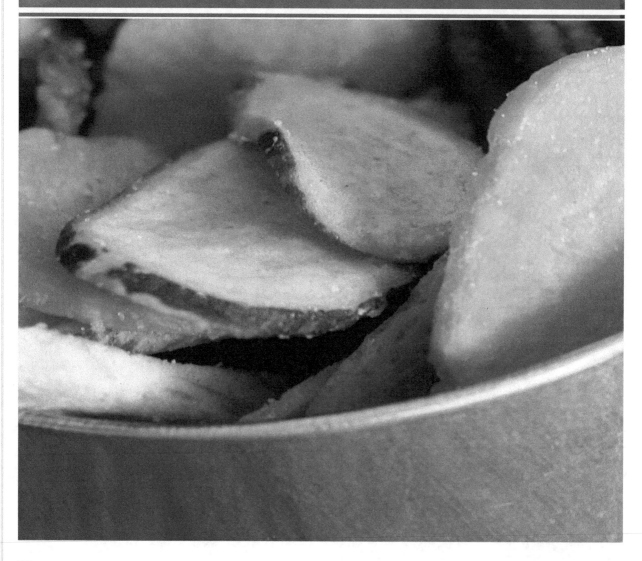

112)   MIXED VEGETABLES WITH BASIL

Preparation Time: 40 minutes

Servings: 4

Ingredients:

- ✓ 2 medium zucchinis, chopped
- ✓ 2 medium yellow squash, chopped
- ✓ 1 red onion, cut into 1-inch wedges
- ✓ 1 red bell pepper, diced
- ✓ 1 cup cherry tomatoes, halved
- ✓ 4 tbsp olive oil
- ✓ Salt and black pepper to taste
- ✓ 3 garlic cloves, minced
- ✓ 2/3 cup whole-wheat breadcrumbs
- ✓ 1 lemon, zested
- ✓ ¼ cup chopped fresh basil

Directions:

- ❖ Preheat the oven to 450 F. Lightly grease a large baking sheet with cooking spray.
- ❖ In a medium bowl, add the zucchini, yellow squash, red onion, bell pepper, tomatoes, olive oil, salt, black pepper, and garlic. Toss well and spread the mixture on the baking sheet. Roast in the oven for 25 to 30 minutes or until the vegetables are tender while stirring every 5 minutes.
- ❖ Meanwhile, heat the olive oil in a medium skillet and sauté the garlic until fragrant. Mix in the breadcrumbs, lemon zest, and basil. Cook for 2 to 3 minutes. Remove the vegetables from the oven and toss in the breadcrumb's mixture. Serve

113)   ONION RINGS AND KALE DIP

Preparation Time: 35 minutes

Servings: 4

Ingredients:

- ✓ 1 onion, sliced into rings
- ✓ 1 tbsp flaxseed meal + 3 tbsp water
- ✓ 1 cup almond flour
- ✓ ½ cup grated plant-based Parmesan
- ✓ 2 tsp garlic powder
- ✓ ½ tbsp sweet paprika powder
- ✓ 2 oz chopped kale
- ✓ 2 tbsp olive oil
- ✓ 2 tbsp dried cilantro
- ✓ 1 tbsp dried oregano
- ✓ Salt and black pepper to taste
- ✓ 1 cup tofu mayonnaise
- ✓ 4 tbsp coconut cream
- ✓ Juice of ½ a lemon

Directions:

- ❖ Preheat oven to 400 F. In a bowl, mix the flaxseed meal and water and leave the mixture to thicken and fully absorb for 5 minutes. In another bowl, combine almond flour, plant-based Parmesan cheese, half of the garlic powder, sweet paprika, and salt. Line a baking sheet with parchment paper in readiness for the rings. When the vegan "flax egg" is ready, dip in the onion rings one after another, and then into the almond flour mixture. Place the rings on the baking sheet and grease with cooking spray. Bake for 15-20 minutes or until golden brown and crispy. Remove the onion rings into a serving bowl.
- ❖ Put kale in a food processor. Add in olive oil, cilantro, oregano, remaining garlic powder, salt, black pepper, tofu mayonnaise, coconut cream, and lemon juice; puree until nice and smooth. Allow the dip to sit for about 10 minutes for the flavors to develop. After, serve the dip with the crispy onion rings

114)   SOY CHORIZO STUFFED CABBAGE ROLLS

Preparation Time: 35 minutes

Servings: 4

Ingredients:

- ✓ ¼ cup coconut oil, divided
- ✓ 1 large white onion, chopped
- ✓ 3 cloves garlic, minced, divided
- ✓ 1 cup crumbled soy chorizo
- ✓ 1 cup cauliflower rice
- ✓ 1 can tomato sauce
- ✓ 1 tsp dried oregano
- ✓ 1 tsp dried basil
- ✓ 8 full green cabbage leaves

Directions:

- ❖ Heat half of the coconut oil in a saucepan over medium heat.
- ❖ Add half of the onion, half of the garlic, and all of the soy chorizo. Sauté for 5 minutes or until the chorizo has browned further, and the onion softened. Stir in the cauli rice, season with salt and black pepper, and cook for 3 to 4 minutes. Turn the heat off and set the pot aside.
- ❖ Heat the remaining oil in a saucepan over medium heat, add, and sauté the remaining onion and garlic until fragrant and soft. Pour in the tomato sauce, and season with salt, black pepper, oregano, and basil. Add ¼ cup water and simmer the sauce for 10 minutes.
- ❖ While the sauce cooks, lay the cabbage leaves on a flat surface and spoon the soy chorizo mixture into the middle of each leaf. Roll the leaves to secure the filling. Place the cabbage rolls in the tomato sauce and cook further for 10 minutes. When ready, serve the cabbage rolls with sauce over mashed broccoli or with mixed seed bread

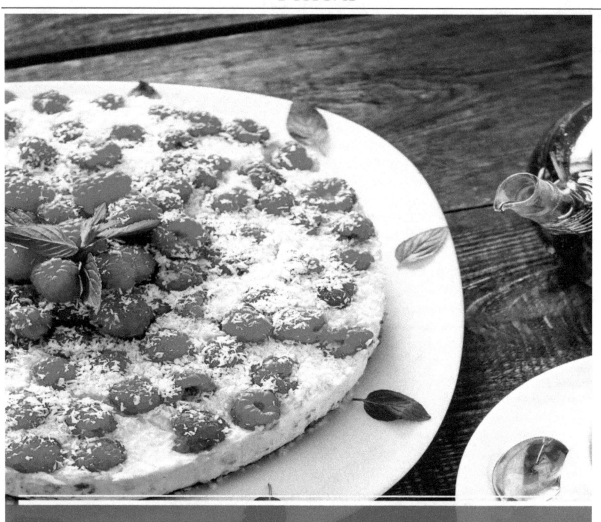

DESSERTS

115)   RAW RASPBERRY CHEESECAKE

Preparation Time: 15 minutes + chilling time   **Servings:** 9

Ingredients:

- ✓ Filling:
- ✓ 2 cups raw cashews, soaked overnight and drained
- ✓ 14 ounces blackberries, frozen
- ✓ 1 tbsp fresh lime juice
- ✓ 1/4 tsp crystallized ginger
- ✓ 1 can coconut cream
- ✓ 8 fresh dates, pitted

- ✓ Crust:
- ✓ 2 cups almonds
- ✓ 1 cup fresh dates, pitted
- ✓ 1/4 tsp ground cinnamon

Directions:

- ❖ In your food processor, blend the crust ingredients until the mixture comes together; press the crust into a lightly oiled springform pan.
- ❖ Then, blend the filling layer until completely smooth. Spoon the filling onto the crust, creating a flat surface with a spatula.
- ❖ Transfer the cake to your freezer for about 3 hours. Store in your freezer.
- ❖ Garnish with organic citrus peel. Enjoy

116)   MINI LEMON TARTS

Preparation Time: 15 minutes + chilling time   **Servings:** 9

Ingredients:

- ✓ 1/2 tsp anise, ground
- ✓ 3 lemons, freshly squeezed
- ✓ 1 cup coconut cream
- ✓ 2 tbsp agave syrup

- ✓ 1 cup cashews
- ✓ 1 cup dates, pitted
- ✓ 1/2 cup coconut flakes

Directions:

- ❖ Brush a muffin tin with a nonstick cooking oil.
- ❖ Blend the cashews, dates, coconut and anise in your food processor or a high-speed blender. Press the crust into the peppered muffin tin.
- ❖ Then, blend the lemon, coconut cream and agave syrup. Spoon the cream into the muffin tin.
- ❖ Store in your freezer. Enjoy

117)   COCONUT BLONDIES WITH RAISINS

Preparation Time: 30 minutes   **Servings:** 9

Ingredients:

- ✓ 3/4 cup vegan butter, softened
- ✓ 1 ½ cups brown sugar
- ✓ 3 tbsp applesauce
- ✓ 1/2 tsp vanilla extract
- ✓ 1/2 tsp ground anise
- ✓ 1 cup raisins, soaked for 15 minutes

- ✓ 1 cup coconut flour
- ✓ 1 cup all-purpose flour
- ✓ 1/2 tsp baking powder
- ✓ 1/4 tsp salt
- ✓ 1 cup desiccated coconut, unsweetened

Directions:

- ❖ Start by preheating your oven to 350 degrees F. Brush a baking pan with a nonstick cooking oil.
- ❖ Thoroughly combine the flour, baking powder, salt and coconut. In another bowl, mix the butter, sugar, applesauce, vanilla and anise. Stir the butter mixture into the dry ingredients; stir to combine well.
- ❖ Fold in the raisins. Press the batter into the prepared baking pan.
- ❖ Bake for approximately 25 minutes or until it is set in the middle. Place the cake on a wire rack to cool slightly.
- ❖ Enjoy

118)   CHOCOLATE SQUARES

Preparation Time: 1 hour 10 minutes   **Servings:** 20

Ingredients:

- ✓ 2 ounces dark chocolate
- ✓ 4 tbsp agave syrup
- ✓ 1 tsp vanilla paste
- ✓ 1/4 tsp ground cinnamon
- ✓ 1/4 tsp ground cloves

- ✓ 1 cup cashew butter
- ✓ 1 cup almond butter
- ✓ 1/4 cup coconut oil, melted
- ✓ 1/4 cup raw cacao powder

Directions:

- ❖ Process all the ingredients in your blender until uniform and smooth.
- ❖ Scrape the batter into a parchment-lined baking sheet. Place it in your freezer for at least 1 hour to set.
- ❖ Cut into squares and serve. Enjoy

119) CHOCOLATE AND RAISIN COOKIE BARS

Preparation Time: 40 minutes

Servings: 10

Ingredients:

- ✓ 1/2 cup peanut butter, at room temperature
- ✓ 1 cup agave syrup
- ✓ 1 tsp pure vanilla extract
- ✓ 1/4 tsp kosher salt
- ✓ 2 cups almond flour
- ✓ 1 tsp baking soda
- ✓ 1 cup raisins
- ✓ 1 cup vegan chocolate, broken into chunks

Directions:

- ❖ In a mixing bowl, thoroughly combine the peanut butter, agave syrup, vanilla and salt.
- ❖ Gradually stir in the almond flour and baking soda and stir to combine. Add in the raisins and chocolate chunks and stir again.
- ❖ Freeze for about 30 minutes and serve well chilled. Enjoy

120) ALMOND GRANOLA BARS

Preparation Time: 25 minutes

Servings: 12

Ingredients:

- ✓ 1/2 cup spelt flour
- ✓ 1/2 cup oat flour
- ✓ 1 cup rolled oats
- ✓ 1 tsp baking powder
- ✓ 1/2 tsp cinnamon
- ✓ 1/2 tsp ground cardamom
- ✓ 1/4 tsp freshly grated nutmeg
- ✓ 1/8 tsp kosher salt
- ✓ 1 cup almond milk
- ✓ 3 tbsp agave syrup
- ✓ 1/2 cup peanut butter
- ✓ 1/2 cup applesauce
- ✓ 1/2 tsp pure almond extract
- ✓ 1/2 tsp pure vanilla extract
- ✓ 1/2 cup almonds, slivered

Directions:

- ❖ Begin by preheating your oven to 350 degrees F.
- ❖ In a mixing bowl, thoroughly combine the flour, oats, baking powder and spices. In another bowl, combine the wet ingredients.
- ❖ Then, stir the wet mixture into the dry ingredients; mix to combine well. Fold in the slivered almonds.
- ❖ Scrape the batter mixture into a parchment-lined baking pan. Bake in the preheated oven for about 20 minutes. Let it cool on a wire rack. Cut into bars and enjoy

121) COCONUT COOKIES

Preparation Time: 40 minutes

Servings: 10

Ingredients:

- ✓ 1/2 cup oat flour
- ✓ 1/2 cup all-purpose flour
- ✓ 1/2 tsp baking soda
- ✓ A pinch of salt
- ✓ 1/4 tsp grated nutmeg
- ✓ 1/2 tsp ground cloves
- ✓ 1/2 tsp ground cinnamon
- ✓ 4 tbsp coconut oil
- ✓ 2 tbsp oat milk
- ✓ 1/2 cup coconut sugar
- ✓ 1/2 cup coconut flakes, unsweetened

Directions:

- ❖ In a mixing bowl, combine the flour, baking soda and spices.
- ❖ In another bowl, combine the coconut oil, oat milk, sugar and coconut. Stir the wet mixture into the dry ingredients and stir until well combined.
- ❖ Place the batter in your refrigerator for about 30 minutes. Shape the batter into small cookies and arrange them on a parchment-lined cookie pan.
- ❖ Bake in the preheated oven at 330 degrees F for approximately 10 minutes. Transfer the pan to a wire rack to cool at room temperature. Enjoy

122) RAW WALNUT AND BERRY CAKE

Preparation Time: 10 minutes + chilling time

Servings: 8

Ingredients:

- ✓ Crust:
- ✓ 1 ½ cups walnuts, ground
- ✓ 2 tbsp maple syrup
- ✓ 1/4 cup raw cacao powder
- ✓ 1/4 tsp ground cinnamon
- ✓ A pinch of coarse salt
- ✓ A pinch of freshly grated nutmeg
- ✓ Berry layer:
- ✓ 6 cups mixed berries
- ✓ 2 frozen bananas
- ✓ 1/2 cup agave syrup

Directions:

- ❖ In your food processor, blend the crust ingredients until the mixture comes together; press the crust into a lightly oiled baking pan.
- ❖ Then, blend the berry layer. Spoon the berry layer onto the crust, creating a flat surface with a spatula.
- ❖ Transfer the cake to your freezer for about 3 hours. Store in your freezer. Enjoy

THE PLANT-BASED DIET FOR ONE

The Revolutionary Recipe Book with Easy and Tasty Recipes for Healthy Lifestyle and Smart People!

Lose Rapidly Weight with a Large Choice of 120+ Vegan and Vegetarian Recipes!

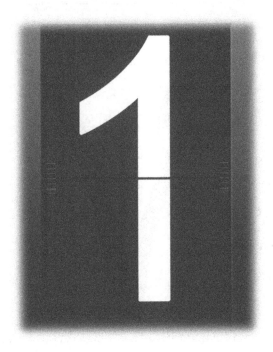

By

Audrey Pottery

TABLE OF CONTENT

PART 2-INTRODUCTION to PLANT-BASED DIET

I've been on a primarily plant-based diet for a couple of years now, and I feel happy, energetic, and full of life. That's why I'm taking this opportunity to share my experiences with you through this cookbook.

This Plant-Based Cookbook comes from a deep place of passion and teaching where I guide those who diet regularly and beginners who want to transition to the plant-based lifestyle on its importance in today's age. It considers a trendy eating style, busy schedules, and tasty ideas to ensure that each recipe produced is not dull but delicious enough to enjoy cooking and eating.

My suggestion is to give the recipes a direct dive and enjoy all the delicious goodness that awaits you.

While the plant-based diet may seem torn between the vegetarian and vegan diets, it is neither. It is not a diet but a healthy lifestyle.

Unsurprisingly, an extensive discussion argues that the plant-based diet is either vegan (which is plant-centric) or vegetarian (which accommodates a certain amount of animal foods). Both cases are incorrect, however. The plant-based diet uses plant-based foods and strongly rejects processed foods such as white rice and added sugars. On the other hand, vegan and vegetarian diets allow some processed foods.

In this book, my goal is to present you with plant-based recipes in their healthiest form. The cookbook seeks to guide you. Beginners to the plant-based diet especially appreciate the essentials of whole plant foods, giving you flexible options and various cooking combinations.

Benefits of the plant-based diet

Plant-based foods are an excellent source of many nutrients that boost the body's metabolism in many ways. In addition, they are easy to digest due to their rich antioxidant content.

- Reduced risk of heart disease

Processed and animal foods are culprits of many heart diseases. The whole plant-based diet is better at nourishing the body with essential nutrients, improving the heart's function of producing and transporting blood to and from various parts of the body.

- Prevents and cures diabetes

Plant-based foods are excellent at reducing high blood sugar. Many studies that compared a vegetarian and vegan diet to a regular meat-filled diet showed that a diet with more plant-based foods reduced the risk of diabetes by 50%.

- An improved cognitive inclination

Fruits and vegetables are excellent for cleansing and increasing metabolism. They release a high number of plant compounds and antioxidants that slow or prevent cognitive decline. On a plant-based diet, the brain is boosted with sustainable energy, promoting sharp memory, language, thinking, and judgment skills.

- Rapid weight loss

A diet high in animal foods is known to promote weight gain. However, switching to a plant-based diet helps the body get rid of fat walls quickly, which results in rapid weight loss.

What to eat in a Plant-Based Lifestyle and PB Swaps

- Fruits - consume a wide range of fruits, whether fresh, dried, boiled, pureed, etc.

- Vegetables - all vegetables are permissible in the plant-based diet. They also provide plenty of essential vitamins and minerals for the body.

- Legumes are an excellent source of plant-based protein and fiber. Fiber is a nutrient that many people lack, and it is essential to increase its content in the body.

- Whole grains provide the body with nutrients such as selenium, copper, and magnesium. Meanwhile, they are rich in fiber when consumed in their whole-grain form. Avoid processed flours, rice, pasta, and bread in your plant-based diet, but consume brown rice, whole-wheat pasta, whole wheat bread, oats, barley, buckwheat, rye, quinoa spelled.

- Walnuts and nut butter - Walnuts are an essential source of selenium, vitamin E, and plant-based protein. They are excellent additions to desserts, smoothies, and snacks.

- Seeds are rich in calcium, vitamins, and healthy fats. Consume chia seeds, hemp seeds, flax seeds, pumpkin seeds, sunflower seeds, sesame seeds, etc.

- Healthy Oils and Fats - Plants offer a few options of healthy, fragrant oils and fats that are perfect for cooking, frying, sautéing, etc. They serve as an excellent substitute for dairy products and are rich in omega-3 fatty acids. Use olive oil, avocado, canola oil, walnuts, peanuts, hemp seeds, flax seeds, chia seeds, cashews, coconut oil.

- Plant-based milk, cream, and cheese - going plant-based doesn't mean staying away from creamy, milky, cheesy foods. You can instead plant-based alternatives using almond milk, soy milk, rice milk, cashew milk, coconut milk, coconut cream, cashew cream, hemp milk, oat milk.

- Plant-based meats - Have tofu, tempeh, seitan.

- Spices, herbs, and seasonings - All plant-based spices, herbs, and seasonings are permissible in the plant-based diet. Use basil example, turmeric, curry, black pepper, rosemary, oregano, thyme, sage, marjoram, salt, salsa, soy sauce, nutritional yeast, vinegar, homemade BBQ sauce, a homemade plant-based mayonnaise, etc.

- Beverages - You can drink coffee, sparkling water, tea, smoothies, etc.

FOOD TO AVOID

It has been established that all animal foods are not allowed in the plant-based diet, but other products are not allowed in a plant-based diet. Here is a detailed list:
- Animal meat: poultry, seafood, pork, lamb, and beef
- Butter, ghee, and other solid animal fats
- All processed foods
- Sugary foods such as cookies, cakes, and pastries
- All refined white carbohydrates
- Processed vegan and vegetarian alternatives that may contain added salt or sugar
- Excessive salt
- Fried foods

EIGHT FOOD-BASED MISTAKES

Without a clear understanding of the diet, people can make some mistakes while following a plant-based diet. This is mainly due to the subtle differences between the ingredients. The following are common food mistakes that people usually make and the different ways to avoid them:

BREAD

There are countless varieties of bread available today. While all loaves are made primarily from a basic flour batter, many additional ingredients can compromise the plant-based diet. The addition of butter, animal milk, fat or other animal products, or an excess of sugar and salt can make bread unsuitable for a plant-based diet. Be sure to double-check the ingredients in store-bought bread or make your bread at home using only vegan ingredients.

BROTH FOR SOUPS

Broths are commonly used in soups and curries, but most are liquid extracts of bones, meat, and vegetables. Because chicken and beef broths are usually used in popular soup recipes, people also use them in a plant-based diet. Vegetable broths and stocks should be used instead. The broth gets most of its nutrients and fat from the meat or bones in which it is cooked, so only vegetable broths are recommended for this diet.

PASTA

Whole wheat or basic flour pasta is an excellent option for enjoying some flavor and variety in your plant-based diet. Adding pasta to your plant-based menu is not harmful, but if the same pasta is cooked with animal ingredients, it is not suitable for this diet. Plant-based pasta recipes, including zucchini spaghetti, are also an excellent option for this diet.

ORANGE JUICE

Freshly squeezed organic orange juice is not nasty for the plant-based diet. It is a good source of vitamin C. However, when the juice is processed to add additional nutrients, the problem begins. Some companies add vitamin D2 or D3 to the juice. While vitamin D2 comes from plants, vitamin D3 is an animal-based vitamin not allowed in a plant-based diet. Read labels and do your research to avoid such products. It's best to rely on homemade, freshly squeezed juices rather than store-bought ones.

GRANOLA
Granola comes in a wide variety. Because of the diversity of ingredients used in different granola recipes, a person on a plant-based diet should be more careful in their selection. Granola may contain dairy products such as milk, butter, or eggs. These should be avoided completely. Instead, choose one made from oats, nuts, seeds, and vegetable fats while following this diet.

CREAMS AND CUSTARDS
Since all creams and cream cheeses are made from animal milk, they are prohibited in a plant-based diet, even in small amounts. Instead, non-dairy, plant-based creams should be used. Ointments made from soy or coconut milk taste good and have a rich, thick texture, just like other creams.

CHEESE
Cheese is a staple in most diets, but they are animal-based and now allowed, as mentioned above. This is where vegan cheeses come in. These cheeses are made with plant-based ingredients, including soy, nuts, tapioca, coconut, root vegetables, or aquafaba. Like dairy cheese, vegan cheese varies in shape, texture, and taste but provides a good substitute for animal-based cheese.

VEGAN SAUSAGES AND BURGERS
Burgers and sausages are commonly enjoyed and hard to pass up. Fortunately, now both burgers and sausages are available in plant-based varieties. These burgers and sausages look more like meat-based burgers and sausages but are made of shredded vegetables and batter. Always opt for these varieties while following a plant-based diet.

BREAKFAST

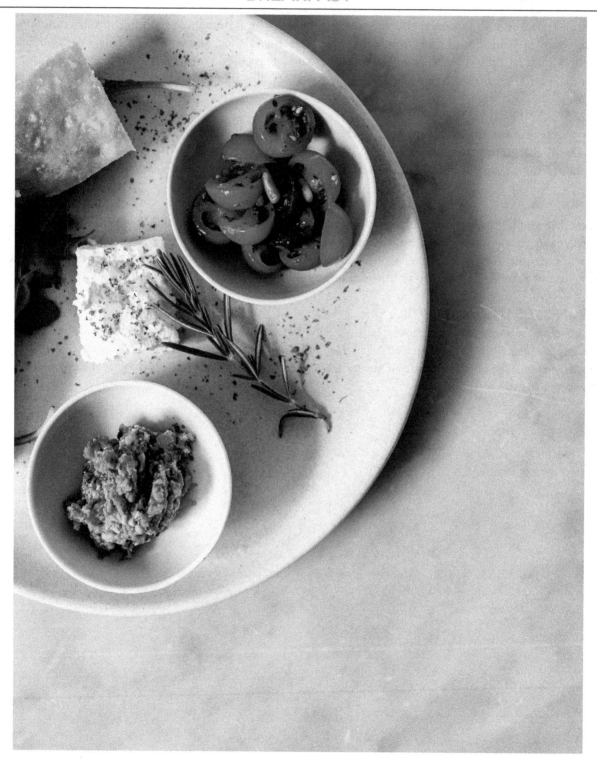

123) BANANA PANCAKES

Preparation Time: 25 minutes

Preparation Time:

Preparation Time: 4

Ingredients:

- ✓ 2 tbsp ground flaxseeds
- ✓ 1/2 cup oat flour
- ✓ 1/2 cup coconut flour
- ✓ 1/2 cup instant oats
- ✓ 1 tsp baking powder
- ✓ 1/4 tsp kosher salt

Ingredients:

- ✓ 1/4 tsp ground cardamom
- ✓ 1/4 tsp ground cinnamon
- ✓ 1/2 tsp coconut extract
- ✓ 1 cup banana
- ✓ 2 tbsp coconut oil, at room temperature

Ingredients:

- ❖ To make the "flax" egg, in a small mixing dish, whisk 2 tbsp of the ground flaxseeds with 4 tbsp of the water. Let it sit for at least 15 minutes.
- ❖ In a mixing bowl, thoroughly combine the flour, oats, baking powder and spices. Add in the flax egg and mashed banana. Mix until everything is well incorporated.
- ❖ Heat 1/2 tbsp of the coconut oil in a frying pan over medium-low flame. Spoon about 1/4 cup of the batter into the frying pan; fry your pancake for approximately 3 minutes per side.
- ❖ Repeat until you run out of batter. Serve with your favorite fixings and enjoy

124) PESTO BREAD

Preparation Time: 35 minutes

Preparation Time:

Preparation Time: 6

Ingredients:

- ✓ 1 ½ cups grated plant-based mozzarella cheese
- ✓ 1 tbsp flax seed powder
- ✓ 4 tbsp coconut flour
- ✓ ½ cup almond flour
- ✓ ½ tsp salt

Ingredients:

- ✓ 1 tsp baking powder
- ✓ 5 tbsp plant butter
- ✓ 2 oz pesto
- ✓ Olive oil for brushing

Ingredients:

- ❖ First, mix the flax seed powder with 3 tbsp water in a bowl, and set aside to soak for 5 minutes.
- ❖ Preheat oven to 350 F and line a baking sheet with parchment paper. In a bowl, evenly combine the coconut flour, almond flour, salt, and baking powder. Melt the plant butter and cheese in a deep skillet over medium heat and stir in the vegan "flax egg." Mix in the flour mixture until a firm dough forms.
- ❖ Turn the heat off, transfer the mixture in between two parchment papers, and then use a rolling pin to flatten out the dough of about an inch's thickness.
- ❖ Remove the parchment paper on top and spread the pesto all over the dough. Now, use a knife to cut the dough into strips, twist each piece, and place it on the baking sheet.
- ❖ Brush with olive oil and bake for 15 to 20 minutes until golden brown.
- ❖ Remove the bread twist; allow cooling for a few minutes, and serve with warm almond milk

125) CLASSIC FRENCH TOASTS

Preparation Time: 16 minutes

Preparation Time:

Preparation Time: 2

Ingredients:

- ✓ 4 tbsp flaxseed
- ✓ 1 tsp plant butter
- ✓ 2 tbsp coconut flour
- ✓ 2 tbsp almond flour
- ✓ 1 ½ tsp baking powder
- ✓ A pinch of salt

Ingredients:

- ✓ 2 tbsp coconut cream
- ✓ 2 tbsp coconut milk whipping cream
- ✓ ½ tsp cinnamon powder
- ✓ 2 tbsp plant butter

Ingredients:

- ❖ For the vegan "flax egg," whisk flax seed powder and 12 tbsp water in two separate bowls and leave to soak for 5 minutes.

- ❖ Grease a glass dish (for the microwave) with 1 tsp plant butter. In another bowl, mix coconut flour, almond flour, baking powder, and salt.

- ❖ When the flaxseed egg is ready, whisk one portion with the coconut cream and add the mixture to the dry ingredients. Continue whisking until the mixture is smooth with no lumps. Pour the dough into the glass dish and microwave for 2 minutes or until the bread's middle part is done. Take out and allow the bread to cool. Remove the bread and slice in half. Return to the glass dish.

- ❖ Whisk the remaining vegan "flax egg" with the coconut milk whipping cream until well combined. Pour the mixture over the bread slices and leave to soak. Turn the bread a few times to soak in as much of the batter. Melt 2 tbsp of the plant butter in a frying pan and fry the bread slices on both sides. Transfer to a serving plate, sprinkle with cinnamon powder and serve

126) **CREAMY BREAD WITH SESAME**
Preparation Time: 40 minutes

Preparation Time:

Preparation Time: 6

Ingredients:

- ✓ 4 tbsp flax seed powder
- ✓ 2/3 cup cashew cream cheese
- ✓ 4 tbsp sesame oil + for brushing
- ✓ 1 cup coconut flour

Ingredients:

- ✓ 2 tbsp psyllium husk powder
- ✓ 1 tsp salt
- ✓ 1 tsp baking powder
- ✓ 1 tbsp sesame seeds

Ingredients:

- ❖ In a bowl, mix the flax seed powder with 1 ½ cups water until smoothly combined and set aside to soak for 5 minutes. Preheat oven to 400 F. When the vegan "flax egg" is ready, beat in the cream cheese and sesame oil until well mixed.

- ❖ Whisk in the coconut flour, psyllium husk powder, salt, and baking powder until adequately blended.

- ❖ Grease a 9 x 5 inches baking tray with cooking spray, and spread the dough in the tray. Allow the mixture to stand for 5 minutes and then brush with some sesame oil.

- ❖ Sprinkle with the sesame seeds and bake the dough for 30 minutes or until golden brown on top and set within. Take out the bread and allow cooling for a few minutes. Slice and serve

127) **DIFFERENT SEEDS BREAD**
Preparation Time: 55 minutes

Preparation Time:

Preparation Time: 6

Ingredients:

- ✓ 3 tbsp ground flax seeds
- ✓ ¾ cup coconut flour
- ✓ 1 cup almond flour
- ✓ 3 tsp baking powder
- ✓ 5 tbsp sesame seeds
- ✓ ½ cup chia seeds
- ✓ 1 tsp ground caraway seeds
- ✓ 1 tsp hemp seeds

Ingredients:

- ✓ ¼ cup psyllium husk powder
- ✓ 1 tsp salt
- ✓ 2/3 cup cashew cream cheese
- ✓ ½ cup melted coconut oil
- ✓ ¾ cup coconut cream
- ✓ 1 tbsp poppy seeds

Ingredients:

- ❖ Preheat oven to 350 F and line a loaf pan with parchment paper.
- ❖ For the vegan "flax egg," whisk flax seed powder with ½ cup of water and let the mixture sit to soak for 5 minutes. In a bowl, evenly combine the coconut flour, almond flour, baking powder, sesame seeds, chia seeds, ground caraway seeds, hemp seeds, psyllium husk powder, and salt.
- ❖ In another bowl, use an electric hand mixer to whisk the cream cheese, coconut oil, coconut whipping cream, and vegan "flax egg." Pour the liquid ingredients into the dry ingredients, and continue whisking with the hand mixer until a dough forms. Transfer the dough to the loaf pan, sprinkle with poppy seeds, and bake in the oven for 45 minutes or until a knife inserted into the bread comes out clean. Remove the parchment paper with the bread, and allow cooling on a rack

128) NAAN BREAD

Preparation Time: 25 minutes

Preparation Time:

Preparation Time: 6

Ingredients:

- ✓ ¾ cup almond flour
- ✓ 2 tbsp psyllium husk powder
- ✓ ½ tsp salt
- ✓ ½ tsp baking powder
- ✓ 1/3 cup olive oil

Ingredients:

- ✓ Plant butter for frying
- ✓ 4 oz plant butter
- ✓ 2 garlic cloves, minced

Ingredients:

- ❖ In a bowl, mix the almond flour, psyllium husk powder, salt, and baking powder.
- ❖ Mix in some olive oil and 2 cups of boiling water to combine the ingredients, like a thick porridge. Stir thoroughly and allow the dough to rise for 5 minutes.
- ❖ Divide the dough into 6 to 8 pieces and mold into balls. Place the balls on parchment paper and flatten with your hands.
- ❖ Melt the plant butter in a frying pan and fry the naan on both sides to have a beautiful, golden color. Transfer the naan to a plate and keep warm in the oven. For the garlic butter, add the remaining plant butter to the frying pan and sauté the garlic until fragrant, about 3 minutes. Pour the garlic butter into a bowl and serve as a dip along with the naan

129) MUSHROOM AND SPINACH CHICKPEA OMELETTE

Preparation Time: 25 minutes

Servings: 4

Ingredients:

- ✓ 1 cup chickpea flour
- ✓ ½ tsp onion powder
- ✓ ½ tsp garlic powder
- ✓ ¼ tsp white pepper
- ✓ 1/3 cup nutritional yeast
- ✓ ½ tsp baking soda
- ✓ 1 green bell pepper, chopped
- ✓ 3 scallions, chopped
- ✓ 1 cup sautéed button mushrooms
- ✓ ½ cup chopped fresh spinach
- ✓ 1 cup halved cherry tomatoes
- ✓ 1 tbsp fresh parsley leaves

Directions:

- ❖ In a medium bowl, mix the chickpea flour, onion powder, garlic powder, white pepper, nutritional yeast, and baking soda until well combined. Heat a medium skillet over medium heat and add a quarter of the batter. Swirl the pan to spread the batter across the pan. Scatter a quarter each of the bell pepper, scallions, mushrooms, and spinach on top and cook until the bottom part of the omelet sets, 1-2 minutes.

- ❖ Carefully flip the omelet and cook the other side until set and golden brown. Transfer the omelet to a plate and make the remaining omelets. Serve the omelet with the tomatoes and garnish with the parsley leaves

130) COCONUT-RASPBERRY PANCAKES

Preparation Time: 25 minutes

Servings: 4

Ingredients:

- ✓ 2 tbsp flax seed powder
- ✓ ½ cup coconut milk
- ✓ ¼ cup fresh raspberries, mashed
- ✓ ½ cup oat flour
- ✓ 1 tsp baking soda
- ✓ A pinch salt
- ✓ 1 tbsp coconut sugar
- ✓ 2 tbsp pure date syrup
- ✓ ½ tsp cinnamon powder
- ✓ 2 tbsp unsweetened coconut flakes
- ✓ 2 tsp plant butter
- ✓ Fresh raspberries for garnishing

Directions:

- ❖ In a medium bowl, mix the flax seed powder with the 6 tbsp water and thicken for 5 minutes. Mix in coconut milk and raspberries. Add the oat flour, baking soda, salt, coconut sugar, date syrup, and cinnamon powder. Fold in the coconut flakes until well combined.

- ❖ Working in batches, melt a quarter of the butter in a non-stick skillet and add ¼ cup of the batter. Cook until set beneath and golden brown, 2 minutes. Flip the pancake and cook on the other side until set and golden brown, 2 minutes. Transfer to a plate and make the remaining pancakes using the rest of the ingredients in the same proportions. Garnish the pancakes with some raspberries and serve warm

131) BLUEBERRY-CHIA PUDDING

Preparation Time: 5 minutes + chilling time

Servings: 2

Ingredients:

- ✓ ¾ cup coconut milk
- ✓ ½ tsp vanilla extract
- ✓ ½ cup blueberries
- ✓ 2 tbsp chia seeds
- ✓ Chopped walnuts to garnish

Directions:

- ❖ In a blender, pour the coconut milk, vanilla extract, and half of the blueberries. Process the ingredients at high speed until the blueberries have incorporated into the liquid.

- ❖ Open the blender and mix in the chia seeds. Share the mixture into two breakfast jars, cover, and refrigerate for 4 hours to allow the mixture to gel. Garnish the pudding with the remaining blueberries and walnuts. Serve immediately

132) **POTATO AND CAULIFLOWER BROWNS**

Preparation Time: 35 minutes   **Servings: 4**

Ingredients:

- ✓ 3 tbsp flax seed powder
- ✓ 2 large potatoes, shredded
- ✓ 1 big head cauliflower, riced
- ✓ ½ white onion, grated
- ✓ Salt and black pepper to taste
- ✓ 4 tbsp plant butter

Directions:

- ❖ In a medium bowl, mix the flaxseed powder and 9 tbsp water. Allow thickening for 5 minutes for the vegan "flax egg." Add the potatoes, cauliflower, onion, salt, and black pepper to the vegan "flax egg" and mix until well combined. Allow sitting for 5 minutes to thicken.
- ❖ Working in batches, melt 1 tbsp of plant butter in a non-stick skillet and add 4 scoops of the hashbrown mixture to the skillet. Make sure to have 1 to 2-inch intervals between each scoop.
- ❖ Use the spoon to flatten the batter and cook until compacted and golden brown on the bottom part, 2 minutes. Flip the hashbrowns and cook further for 2 minutes or until the vegetable cook and is golden brown. Transfer to a paper-towel-lined plate to drain grease. Make the remaining hashbrowns using the remaining ingredients. Serve warm

133) PISTACHIOS-PUMPKIN CAKE

Preparation Time: 70 minutes

Servings: 4

Ingredients:

- ✓ 2 tbsp flaxseed powder
- ✓ 3 tbsp vegetable oil
- ✓ ¾ cup canned pumpkin puree
- ✓ ½ cup pure corn syrup
- ✓ 3 tbsp pure date sugar
- ✓ 1 ½ cups whole-wheat flour
- ✓ ½ tsp cinnamon powder
- ✓ ½ tsp baking powder
- ✓ ¼ tsp cloves powder
- ✓ ½ tsp allspice powder
- ✓ ½ tsp nutmeg powder
- ✓ 2 tbsp chopped pistachios

Directions:

- ❖ Preheat the oven to 350 F and lightly coat an 8 x 4-inch loaf pan with cooking spray. In a bowl, mix the flax seed powder with 6 tbsp water and allow thickening for 5 minutes to make the vegan "flax egg."
- ❖ In a bowl, whisk the vegetable oil, pumpkin puree, corn syrup, date sugar, and vegan "flax egg." In another bowl, mix the flour, cinnamon powder, baking powder, cloves powder, allspice powder, and nutmeg powder. Add this mixture to the wet batter and mix until well combined. Pour the batter into the loaf pan, sprinkle the pistachios on top, and gently press the nuts onto the batter to stick.
- ❖ Bake in the oven for 50-55 minutes or until a toothpick inserted into the cake comes out clean. Remove the cake onto a wire rack, allow cooling, slice, and serve

134) BELL PEPPER WITH SCRAMBLED TOFU

Preparation Time: 20 minutes

Servings: 4

Ingredients:

- ✓ 2 tbsp plant butter, for frying
- ✓ 1 (14 oz) pack firm tofu, crumbled
- ✓ 1 red bell pepper, chopped
- ✓ 1 green bell pepper, chopped
- ✓ 1 tomato, finely chopped
- ✓ 2 tbsp chopped fresh green onions
- ✓ Salt and black pepper to taste
- ✓ 1 tsp turmeric powder
- ✓ 1 tsp Creole seasoning
- ✓ ½ cup chopped baby kale
- ✓ ¼ cup grated plant-based Parmesan

Directions:

- ❖ Melt the plant butter in a skillet over medium heat and add the tofu. Cook with occasional stirring until the tofu is light golden brown while, making sure not to break the tofu into tiny bits but to have scrambled egg resemblance, 5 minutes.
- ❖ Stir in the bell peppers, tomato, green onions, salt, black pepper, turmeric powder, and Creole seasoning. Sauté until the vegetables soften, 5 minutes. Mix in the kale to wilt, 3 minutes and then half of the plant-based Parmesan cheese.
- ❖ Allow melting for 1 to 2 minutes and then turn the heat off. Top with the remaining cheese and serve warm

135) ORIGINAL FRENCH TOAST

Preparation Time: 20 minutes

Servings: 2

Ingredients:

- ✓ 1 tbsp ground flax seeds
- ✓ 1 cup coconut milk
- ✓ 1/2 tsp vanilla paste
- ✓ A pinch of sea salt
- ✓ A pinch of grated nutmeg
- ✓ 1/2 tsp ground cinnamon
- ✓ 1/4 tsp ground cloves
- ✓ 1 tbsp agave syrup
- ✓ 4 slices bread

Directions:

- ❖ In a mixing bowl, thoroughly combine the flax seeds, coconut milk, vanilla, salt, nutmeg, cinnamon, cloves and agave syrup.
- ❖ Dredge each slice of bread into the milk mixture until well coated on all sides.
- ❖ Preheat an electric griddle to medium heat and lightly oil it with a nonstick cooking spray.
- ❖ Cook each slice of bread on the preheated griddle for about 3 minutes per side until golden brown.
- ❖ Enjoy

136) FRYBREAD WITH PEANUT BUTTER AND JAM

Preparation Time: 20 minutes

Servings: 3

Ingredients:

- ✓ 1 cup all-purpose flour
- ✓ 1/2 tsp baking powder
- ✓ 1/2 tsp sea salt
- ✓ 1 tsp coconut sugar
- ✓ 1/2 cup warm water
- ✓ 3 tsp olive oil
- ✓ 3 tbsp peanut butter
- ✓ 3 tbsp raspberry jam

Directions:

- ❖ Thoroughly combine the flour, baking powder, salt and sugar. Gradually add in the water until the dough comes together.
- ❖ Divide the dough into three balls; flatten each ball to create circles.
- ❖ Heat 1 tsp of the olive oil in a frying pan over a moderate flame. Fry the first bread for about 9 minutes or until golden brown. Repeat with the remaining oil and dough.
- ❖ Serve the frybread with the peanut butter and raspberry jam. Enjoy

137)   PUDDING WITH SULTANAS ON CIABATTA BREAD

Preparation Time: 2 hours 10 minutes

Servings: 4

Ingredients:

- ✓ 2 cups coconut milk, unsweetened
- ✓ 1/2 cup agave syrup
- ✓ 1 tbsp coconut oil
- ✓ 1/2 tsp vanilla essence
- ✓ 1/2 tsp ground cardamom
- ✓ 1/4 tsp ground cloves
- ✓ 1/2 tsp ground cinnamon
- ✓ 1/4 tsp Himalayan salt
- ✓ 3/4 pound stale ciabatta bread, cubed
- ✓ 1/2 cup sultana raisins

Directions:

- ❖ In a mixing bowl, combine the coconut milk, agave syrup, coconut oil, vanilla, cardamom, ground cloves, cinnamon and Himalayan salt.
- ❖ Add the bread cubes to the custard mixture and stir to combine well. Fold in the sultana raisins and allow it to rest for about 1 hour on a counter.
- ❖ Then, spoon the mixture into a lightly oiled casserole dish.
- ❖ Bake in the preheated oven at 350 degrees F for about 1 hour or until the top is golden brown.
- ❖ Place the bread pudding on a wire rack for 10 minutes before slicing and serving

138)   VEGAN BANH MI

Preparation Time: 35 minutes

Servings: 4

Ingredients:

- ✓ 1/2 cup rice vinegar
- ✓ 1/4 cup water
- ✓ 1/4 cup white sugar
- ✓ 2 carrots, cut into 1/16-inch-thick matchsticks
- ✓ 1/2 cup white (daikon) radish, cut into 1/16-inch-thick matchsticks
- ✓ 1 white onion, thinly sliced
- ✓ 2 tbsp olive oil
- ✓ 12 ounces firm tofu, cut into sticks
- ✓ 1/4 cup vegan mayonnaise
- ✓ 1 ½ tbsp soy sauce
- ✓ 2 cloves garlic, minced
- ✓ 1/4 cup fresh parsley, chopped
- ✓ Kosher salt and ground black pepper, to taste
- ✓ 2 standard French baguettes, cut into four pieces
- ✓ 4 tbsp fresh cilantro, chopped
- ✓ 4 lime wedges

Directions:

- ❖ Bring the rice vinegar, water and sugar to a boil and stir until the sugar has dissolved, about 1 minute. Allow it to cool.
- ❖ Pour the cooled vinegar mixture over the carrot, daikon radish and onion; allow the vegetables to marinate for at least 30 minutes.
- ❖ While the vegetables are marinating, heat the olive oil in a frying pan over medium-high heat. Once hot, add the tofu and sauté for 8 minutes, stirring occasionally to promote even cooking.
- ❖ Then, mix the mayo, soy sauce, garlic, parsley, salt and ground black pepper in a small bowl.
- ❖ Slice each piece of the baguette in half the long way Then, toast the baguette halves under the preheated broiler for about 3 minutes.
- ❖ To assemble the banh mi sandwiches, spread each half of the toasted baguette with the mayonnaise mixture; fill the cavity of the bottom half of the bread with the fried tofu sticks, marinated vegetables and cilantro leaves.
- ❖ Lastly, squeeze the lime wedges over the filling and top with the other half of the baguette. Enjoy

139)   BREAKFAST NUTTY OATMEAL MUFFINS

Preparation Time: 30 minutes

Servings: 9

Ingredients:

- ✓ 1 ½ cups rolled oats
- ✓ 1/2 cup shredded coconut, unsweetened
- ✓ 3/4 tsp baking powder
- ✓ 1/4 tsp salt
- ✓ 1/4 tsp vanilla extract
- ✓ 1/4 tsp coconut extract
- ✓ 1/4 tsp grated nutmeg
- ✓ 1/2 tsp cardamom
- ✓ 3/4 cup coconut milk
- ✓ 1/3 cup canned pumpkin
- ✓ 1/4 cup agave syrup
- ✓ 1/4 cup golden raisins
- ✓ 1/4 cup pecans, chopped

Directions:

- ❖ Begin by preheating your oven to 360 degrees F. Spritz a muffin tin with a nonstick cooking oil.
- ❖ In a mixing bowl, thoroughly combine all the ingredients, except for the raisins and pecans.
- ❖ Fold in the raisins and pecans and scrape the batter into the prepared muffin tin.
- ❖ Bake your muffins for about 25 minutes or until the top is set. Enjoy

140) SMOOTHIE BOWL OF RASPBERRY AND CHIA

Preparation Time: 10 minutes   **Servings:** 2

Ingredients:

- ✓ 1 cup coconut milk
- ✓ 2 small-sized bananas, peeled
- ✓ 1 ½ cups raspberries, fresh or frozen
- ✓ 2 dates, pitted
- ✓ 1 tbsp coconut flakes
- ✓ 1 tbsp pepitas
- ✓ 2 tbsp chia seeds

Directions:

- ❖ In your blender or food processor, mix the coconut milk with the bananas, raspberries and dates.
- ❖ Process until creamy and smooth. Divide the smoothie between two bowls.
- ❖ Top each smoothie bowl with the coconut flakes, pepitas and chia seeds. Enjoy

141) BREAKFAST OATS WITH WALNUTS AND CURRANTS

Preparation Time: 10 minutes   **Servings:** 2

Ingredients:

- ✓ 1 cup water
- ✓ 1 ½ cups oat milk
- ✓ 1 ½ cups rolled oats
- ✓ A pinch of salt
- ✓ A pinch of grated nutmeg
- ✓ 1/4 tsp cardamom
- ✓ 1 handful walnuts, roughly chopped
- ✓ 4 tbsp dried currants

Directions:

- ❖ In a deep saucepan, bring the water and milk to a rolling boil. Add in the oats, cover the saucepan and turn the heat to medium.
- ❖ Add in the salt, nutmeg and cardamom. Continue to cook for about 12 to 13 minutes more, stirring occasionally.
- ❖ Spoon the mixture into serving bowls; top with walnuts and currants. Enjoy

142) APPLESAUCE PANCAKES WITH COCONUT

Preparation Time: 50 minutes   **Servings:** 8

Ingredients:

- ✓ 1 ¼ cups whole-wheat flour
- ✓ 1 tsp baking powder
- ✓ 1/4 tsp sea salt
- ✓ 1/2 tsp ground cinnamon
- ✓ 3/4 cup oat milk
- ✓ 1/2 cup applesauce, unsweetened
- ✓ 2 tbsp coconut oil

Directions:

- ❖ In a mixing bowl, thoroughly combine the flour, baking powder, salt, sugar and spices. Gradually add in the milk and applesauce.
- ❖ Heat a frying pan over a moderately high flame and add a small amount of the coconut oil.

- ✓ 1/2 tsp coconut sugar
- ✓ 1/4 tsp ground cloves
- ✓ 1/4 tsp ground cardamom
- ✓ 8 tbsp coconut, shredded
- ✓ 8 tbsp pure maple syrup

- ❖ Once hot, pour the batter into the frying pan. Cook for approximately 3 minutes until the bubbles form; flip it and cook on the other side for 3 minutes longer until browned on the underside. Repeat with the remaining oil and batter.
- ❖ Serve with shredded coconut and maple syrup. Enjoy

143) VEGGIE PANINI

Preparation Time: 30 minutes

Servings: 4

Ingredients:

- ✓ 1 tbsp olive oil
- ✓ 1 cup sliced button mushrooms
- ✓ Salt and black pepper to taste
- ✓ 1 ripe avocado, sliced
- ✓ 2 tbsp freshly squeezed lemon juice
- ✓ 1 tbsp chopped parsley
- ✓ ½ tsp pure maple syrup
- ✓ 8 slices whole-wheat ciabatta
- ✓ 4 oz sliced plant-based Parmesan

Directions:

- ❖ Heat the olive oil in a medium skillet over medium heat and sauté the mushrooms until softened, 5 minutes. Season with salt and black pepper. Turn the heat off.
- ❖ Preheat a panini press to medium heat, 3 to 5 minutes. Mash the avocado in a medium bowl and mix in the lemon juice, parsley, and maple syrup. Spread the mixture on 4 bread slices, divide the mushrooms and plant-based Parmesan cheese on top.
- ❖ Cover with the other bread slices and brush the top with olive oil. Grill the sandwiches one after another in the heated press until golden brown, and the cheese is melted.
- ❖ Serve

144) **CHEDDAR GRITS AND SOY CHORIZO**

Preparation Time: 25 minutes   **Servings: 6**

Ingredients:

- ✓ 1 cup quick-cooking grits
- ✓ ½ cup grated plant-based cheddar
- ✓ 2 tbsp peanut butter
- ✓ 1 cup soy chorizo, chopped
- ✓ 1 cup corn kernels
- ✓ 2 cups vegetable broth

Directions:

- ❖ Preheat oven to 380 F.
- ❖ Pour the broth in a pot and bring to a boil over medium heat. Stir in salt and grits. Lower the heat and cook until the grits are thickened, stirring often. Turn the heat off, put in the plant-based cheddar cheese, peanut butter, soy chorizo, and corn and mix well.
- ❖ Spread the mixture into a greased baking dish and bake for 45 minutes until slightly puffed and golden brown. Serve right away

145) **VANILLA CREPES AND BERRY CREAM COMPOTE TOPPING**

Preparation Time: 35 minutes   **Servings: 4**

Ingredients:

- ✓ For the berry cream:
- ✓ 2 tbsp plant butter
- ✓ 2 tbsp pure date sugar
- ✓ 1 tsp vanilla extract
- ✓ ½ cup fresh blueberries
- ✓ ½ cup fresh raspberries
- ✓ ½ cup whipped coconut cream
- ✓ For the crepes:
- ✓ 2 tbsp flax seed powder
- ✓ 1 tsp vanilla extract
- ✓ 1 tsp pure date sugar
- ✓ ¼ tsp salt
- ✓ 2 cups almond flour
- ✓ 1 ½ cups almond milk
- ✓ 1 ½ cups water
- ✓ 3 tbsp plant butter for frying

Directions:

- ❖ Melt butter in a pot over low heat and mix in the date sugar, and vanilla. Cook until the sugar melts and then toss in berries. Allow softening for 2-3 minutes. Set aside to cool.
- ❖ In a medium bowl, mix the flax seed powder with 6 tbsp water and allow to thicken for 5 minutes to make the vegan "flax egg." Whisk in vanilla, date sugar, and salt. Pour in a quarter cup of almond flour and whisk, then a quarter cup of almond milk, and mix until no lumps remain. Repeat the mixing process with the remaining almond flour and almond milk in the same quantities until exhausted.
- ❖ Mix in 1 cup of water until the mixture is runny like that of pancakes and add the remaining water until it is lighter. Brush a large non-stick skillet with some butter and place over medium heat to melt. Pour 1 tbsp of the batter into the pan and swirl the skillet quickly and all around to coat the pan with the batter. Cook until the batter is dry and golden brown beneath, about 30 seconds.
- ❖ Use a spatula to carefully flip the crepe and cook the other side until golden brown too. Fold the crepe onto a plate and set aside. Repeat making more crepes with the remaining batter until exhausted. Plate the crepes, top with the whipped coconut cream and the berry compote. Serve immediately

146) STRAWBERRY AND PECAN BREAKFAST

Preparation Time: 15 minutes

Servings: 2

Ingredients:

- ✓ 1 (14-oz) can coconut milk, refrigerated overnight
- ✓ 1 cup granola
- ✓ ½ cup pecans, chopped
- ✓ 1 cup sliced strawberries

Directions:

- ❖ Drain the coconut milk liquid. Layer the coconut milk solids, granola, and strawberries in small glasses. Top with chopped pecans and serve right away

147) GRANOLA WITH HAZELNUTS AND ORANGE

Preparation Time: 50 minutes

Servings: 5

Ingredients:

- ✓ 2 cups rolled oats
- ✓ ¾ cup whole-wheat flour
- ✓ 1 tbsp ground cinnamon
- ✓ 1 tsp ground ginger
- ✓ ½ cup sunflower seeds
- ✓ ½ cup hazelnuts, chopped
- ✓ ½ cup pumpkin seeds
- ✓ ½ cup shredded coconut
- ✓ 1 ¼ cups orange juice
- ✓ ½ cup dried cherries
- ✓ ½ cup goji berries

Directions:

- ❖ Preheat oven to 350 F.
- ❖ In a bowl, combine the oats, flour, cinnamon, ginger, sunflower seeds, hazelnuts, pumpkin seeds, and coconut. Pour in the orange juice, toss to mix well.
- ❖ Transfer to a baking sheet and bake for 15 minutes. Turn the granola and continue baking until it is crunchy, about 30 minutes. Stir in the cherries and goji berries and store in the fridge for up to 14 days

148)   ORANGE CREPES

Preparation Time: 30 minutes   **Servings: 4**

Ingredients:

- ✓ 2 tbsp flax seed powder
- ✓ 1 tsp vanilla extract
- ✓ 1 tsp pure date sugar
- ✓ ¼ tsp salt
- ✓ 2 cups almond flour
- ✓ 1 ½ cups oat milk
- ✓ ½ cup melted plant butter
- ✓ 3 tbsp fresh orange juice
- ✓ 3 tbsp plant butter for frying

Directions:

- ❖ In a medium bowl, mix the flax seed powder with 6 tbsp water and allow thickening for 5 minutes to make the vegan "flax egg." Whisk in the vanilla, date sugar, and salt.
- ❖ Pour in a quarter cup of almond flour and whisk, then a quarter cup of oat milk, and mix until no lumps remain. Repeat the mixing process with the remaining almond flour and almond milk in the same quantities until exhausted.
- ❖ Mix in the plant butter, orange juice, and half of the water until the mixture is runny like pancakes. Add the remaining water until the mixture is lighter. Brush a non-stick skillet with some butter and place over medium heat to melt.
- ❖ Pour 1 tbsp of the batter into the pan and swirl the skillet quickly and all around to coat the pan with the batter. Cook until the batter is dry and golden brown beneath, about 30 seconds.
- ❖ Use a spatula to flip the crepe and cook the other side until golden brown too. Fold the crepe onto a plate and set aside. Repeat making more crepes with the remaining batter until exhausted. Drizzle some maple syrup on the crepes and serve

149)   OAT BREAD WITH COCONUT

Preparation Time: 50 minutes   **Servings: 4**

Ingredients:

- ✓ 4 cups whole-wheat flour
- ✓ ¼ tsp salt
- ✓ ½ cup rolled oats
- ✓ 1 tsp baking soda
- ✓ 1 ¾ cups coconut milk, thick
- ✓ 2 tbsp pure maple syrup

Directions:

- ❖ Preheat the oven to 400 F.
- ❖ In a bowl, mix flour, salt, oats, and baking soda. Add in coconut milk and maple syrup and whisk until dough forms. Dust your hands with some flour and knead the dough into a ball. Shape the dough into a circle and place on a baking sheet.
- ❖ Cut a deep cross on the dough and bake in the oven for 15 minutes at 450 F. Reduce the temperature to 400 F and bake further for 20 to 25 minutes or until a hollow sound is made when the bottom of the bread is tapped. Slice and serve

150)   BOWL WITH BLACK BEANS AND SPICY QUINOA

Preparation Time: 25 minutes   **Servings: 4**

Ingredients:

- ✓ 1 cup brown quinoa, rinsed
- ✓ 3 tbsp plant-based yogurt
- ✓ ½ lime, juiced
- ✓ 2 tbsp chopped fresh cilantro
- ✓ 1 (5 oz) can black beans, drained
- ✓ 3 tbsp tomato salsa
- ✓ ¼ avocado, sliced
- ✓ 2 radishes, shredded
- ✓ 1 tbsp pepitas (pumpkin seeds)

Directions:

- ❖ Cook the quinoa with 2 cups of slightly salted water in a medium pot over medium heat or until the liquid absorbs, 15 minutes. Spoon the quinoa into serving bowls and fluff with a fork.
- ❖ In a small bowl, mix the yogurt, lime juice, cilantro, and salt. Divide this mixture on the quinoa and top with the beans, salsa, avocado, radishes, and pepitas. Serve immediately

151) ALMOND AND RAISIN GRANOLA

Preparation Time: 20 minutes

Servings: 8

Ingredients:

- ✓ 5 ½ cups old-fashioned oats
- ✓ 1 ½ cups chopped walnuts
- ✓ ½ cup shelled sunflower seeds
- ✓ 1 cup golden raisins
- ✓ 1 cup shaved almonds
- ✓ 1 cup pure maple syrup
- ✓ ½ tsp ground cinnamon
- ✓ ¼ tsp ground allspice
- ✓ A pinch of salt

Directions:

- ❖ Preheat oven to 325 F. In a baking dish, place the oats, walnuts, and sunflower seeds. Bake for 10 minutes.
- ❖ Lower the heat from the oven to 300 F. Stir in the raisins, almonds, maple syrup, cinnamon, allspice, and salt. Bake for an additional 15 minutes. Allow cooling before serving

152) PECAN AND PUMPKIN SEED OAT JARS

Preparation Time: 10 minutes + chilling time

Servings: 5

Ingredients:

- ✓ 2 ½ cups old-fashioned rolled oats
- ✓ 5 tbsp pumpkin seeds
- ✓ 5 tbsp chopped pecans
- ✓ 5 cups unsweetened soy milk
- ✓ 2 ½ tsp agave syrup
- ✓ Salt to taste
- ✓ 1 tsp ground cardamom
- ✓ 1 tsp ground ginger

Directions:

- ❖ • In a bowl, put oats, pumpkin seeds, pecans, soy milk, agave syrup, salt, cardamom, and ginger and toss to combine. Divide the mixture between mason jars. Seal the lids and transfer to the fridge to soak for 10-12 hours

153) EASY APPLE MUFFINS

Preparation Time: 40 minutes

Servings: 4

Ingredients:

- ✓ For the muffins:
- ✓ 1 flax seed powder + 3 tbsp water
- ✓ 1 ½ cups whole-wheat
- ✓ For topping:
- ✓ 1/3 cup whole-wheat flour
- ✓ ½ cup pure date sugar

Directions:

- ❖ Preheat oven to 400 F and grease 6 muffin cups with cooking spray. In a bowl, mix the flax seed powder with water and allow thickening for 5 minutes to make the vegan "flax egg."

flour

- ✓ ¾ cup pure date sugar
- ✓ 2 tsp baking powder
- ✓ ¼ tsp salt
- ✓ 1 tsp cinnamon powder
- ✓ 1/3 cup melted plant butter
- ✓ 1/3 cup flax milk
- ✓ 2 apples, chopped

- ✓ ½ cup cold plant butter, cubed
- ✓ 1 ½ tsp cinnamon powder

❖ In a bowl, mix flour, date sugar, baking powder, salt, and cinnamon powder. Whisk in the butter, vegan "flax egg," flax milk, and fold in the apples. Fill the muffin cups two-thirds way up with the batter.

❖ In a bowl, mix remaining flour, date sugar, cold butter, and cinnamon powder. Sprinkle the mixture on the muffin batter. Bake for 20 minutes. Remove the muffins onto a wire rack, allow cooling, and serve

154) ALMOND YOGURT WITH BERRIES AND WALNUTS

Preparation Time: 10 minutes   **Servings: 4**

Ingredients:

- ✓ 4 cups almond milk
- ✓ Dairy-Free yogurt, cold
- ✓ 2 tbsp pure malt syrup

- ✓ 2 cups mixed berries, chopped
- ✓ ¼ cup chopped toasted walnuts

Directions:

❖ In a medium bowl, mix the yogurt and malt syrup until well-combined. Divide the mixture into 4 breakfast bowls. Top with the berries and walnuts. Enjoy immediately

155) BREAKFAST BLUEBERRY MUESLI

Preparation Time: 10 minutes   **Servings: 5**

Ingredients:

- ✓ 2 cups spelt flakes
- ✓ 2 cups puffed cereal
- ✓ ¼ cup sunflower seeds
- ✓ ¼ cup almonds
- ✓ ¼ cup raisins
- ✓ ¼ cup dried cranberries

- ✓ ¼ cup chopped dried figs
- ✓ ¼ cup shredded coconut
- ✓ ¼ cup non-dairy chocolate chips
- ✓ 3 tsp ground cinnamon
- ✓ ½ cup coconut milk
- ✓ ½ cup blueberries

Directions:

❖ • In a bowl, combine the spelt flakes, puffed cereal, sunflower seeds, almonds, raisins, cranberries, figs, coconut, chocolate chips, and cinnamon. Toss to mix well. Pour in the coconut milk. Let sit for 1 hour and serve topped with blueberries

156) **BERRY AND ALMOND BUTTER SWIRL BOWL**

Preparation Time: 10 minutes   **Servings: 3**

Ingredients:

- ✓ 1 ½ cups almond milk
- ✓ 2 small bananas
- ✓ 2 cups mixed berries, fresh or frozen
- ✓ 3 dates, pitted
- ✓ 3 scoops hemp protein powder
- ✓ 3 tbsp smooth almond butter
- ✓ 2 tbsp pepitas

Directions:

- ❖ In your blender or food processor, mix the almond milk with the bananas, berries and dates.
- ❖ Process until everything is well combined. Divide the smoothie between three bowls.
- ❖ Top each smoothie bowl with almond butter and use a butter knife to swirl the almond butter into the top of each smoothie bowl.
- ❖ Afterwards, garnish each smoothie bowl with pepitas, serve well-chilled and enjoy

157) **OATS WITH COCONUT AND STRAWBERRIES**

Preparation Time: 15 minutes   **Servings: 2**

Ingredients:

- ✓ 1/2 tbsp coconut oil
- ✓ 1 cup rolled oats
- ✓ A pinch of flaky sea salt
- ✓ 1/8 tsp grated nutmeg
- ✓ 1/4 tsp cardamom
- ✓ 1 tbsp coconut sugar
- ✓ 1 cup coconut milk, sweetened
- ✓ 1 cup water
- ✓ 2 tbsp coconut flakes
- ✓ 4 tbsp fresh strawberries

Directions:

- ❖ In a saucepan, melt the coconut oil over a moderate flame. Then, toast the oats for about 3 minutes, stirring continuously.
- ❖ Add in the salt, nutmeg, cardamom, coconut sugar, milk and water; continue to cook for 12 minutes more or until cooked through.
- ❖ Spoon the mixture into serving bowls; top with coconut flakes and fresh strawberries. Enjoy

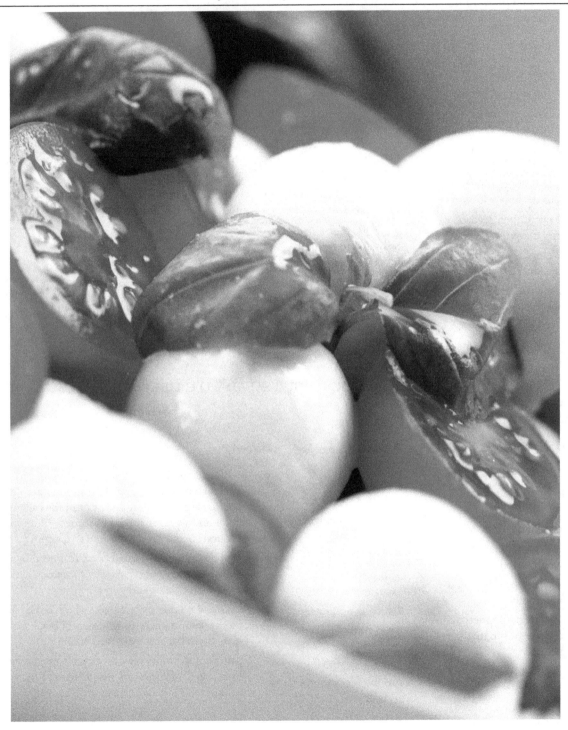

158) BLACK BEAN QUINOA SALAD

Preparation Time: 15 minutes + chilling time

Servings: 4

Ingredients:

- ✓ 2 cups water
- ✓ 1 cup quinoa, rinsed
- ✓ 16 ounces canned black beans, drained
- ✓ 2 Roma tomatoes, sliced
- ✓ 1 red onion, thinly sliced
- ✓ 1 cucumber, seeded and chopped
- ✓ 2 cloves garlic, pressed or minced
- ✓ 2 Italian peppers, seeded and sliced
- ✓ 2 tbsp fresh parsley, chopped
- ✓ 2 tbsp fresh cilantro, chopped
- ✓ 1/4 cup olive oil
- ✓ 1 lemon, freshly squeezed
- ✓ 1 tbsp apple cider vinegar
- ✓ 1/2 tsp dried dill weed
- ✓ 1/2 tsp dried oregano
- ✓ Sea salt and ground black pepper, to taste

Directions:

- ❖ Place the water and quinoa in a saucepan and bring it to a rolling boil. Immediately turn the heat to a simmer.
- ❖ Let it simmer for about 13 minutes until the quinoa has absorbed all of the water; fluff the quinoa with a fork and let it cool completely. Then, transfer the quinoa to a salad bowl.
- ❖ Add the remaining ingredients to the salad bowl and toss to combine well. Enjoy

159) POWER BULGUR SALAD WITH HERBS

Preparation Time: 20 minutes + chilling time

Servings: 4

Ingredients:

- ✓ 2 cups water
- ✓ 1 cup bulgur
- ✓ 12 ounces canned chickpeas, drained
- ✓ 1 Persian cucumber, thinly sliced
- ✓ 2 bell peppers, seeded and thinly sliced
- ✓ 1 jalapeno pepper, seeded and thinly sliced
- ✓ 2 Roma tomatoes, sliced
- ✓ 1 onion, thinly sliced
- ✓ 2 tbsp fresh basil, chopped
- ✓ 2 tbsp fresh parsley, chopped
- ✓ 2 tbsp fresh mint, chopped
- ✓ 2 tbsp fresh chives, chopped
- ✓ 4 tbsp olive oil
- ✓ 1 tbsp balsamic vinegar
- ✓ 1 tbsp lemon juice
- ✓ 1 tsp fresh garlic, pressed
- ✓ Sea salt and freshly ground black pepper, to taste
- ✓ 2 tbsp nutritional yeast
- ✓ 1/2 cup Kalamata olives, sliced

Directions:

- ❖ In a saucepan, bring the water and bulgur to a boil. Immediately turn the heat to a simmer and let it cook for about 20 minutes or until the bulgur is tender and water is almost absorbed. Fluff with a fork and spread on a large tray to let cool.
- ❖ Place the bulgur in a salad bowl followed by the chickpeas, cucumber, peppers, tomatoes, onion, basil, parsley, mint and chives.
- ❖ In a small mixing dish, whisk the olive oil, balsamic vinegar, lemon juice, garlic, salt and black pepper. Dress the salad and toss to combine.
- ❖ Sprinkle nutritional yeast over the top, garnish with olives and serve at room temperature. Enjoy

160) ORIGINAL ROASTED PEPPER SALAD

Preparation Time: 15 minutes + chilling time

Servings: 3

Ingredients:

- ✓ 6 bell peppers
- ✓ 3 tbsp extra-virgin olive oil
- ✓ 3 tsp red wine vinegar
- ✓ 3 garlic cloves, finely chopped
- ✓ 2 tbsp fresh parsley, chopped
- ✓ Sea salt and freshly cracked black pepper, to taste
- ✓ 1/2 tsp red pepper flakes
- ✓ 6 tbsp pine nuts, roughly chopped

Directions:

- ❖ Broil the peppers on a parchment-lined baking sheet for about 10 minutes, rotating the pan halfway through the cooking time, until they are charred on all sides.
- ❖ Then, cover the peppers with a plastic wrap to steam. Discard the skin, seeds and cores.
- ❖ Slice the peppers into strips and toss them with the remaining ingredients. Place in your refrigerator until ready to serve. Enjoy

161) WINTER HEARTY QUINOA SOUP

Preparation Time: 25 minutes

Servings: 4

Ingredients:

- ✓ 2 tbsp olive oil
- ✓ 1 onion, chopped
- ✓ 2 carrots, peeled and chopped
- ✓ 1 parsnip, chopped
- ✓ 1 celery stalk, chopped
- ✓ 1 cup yellow squash, chopped
- ✓ 4 garlic cloves, pressed or minced
- ✓ 4 cups roasted vegetable broth
- ✓ 2 medium tomatoes, crushed
- ✓ 1 cup quinoa
- ✓ Sea salt and ground black pepper, to taste
- ✓ 1 bay laurel
- ✓ 2 cup Swiss chard, tough ribs removed and torn into pieces
- ✓ 2 tbsp Italian parsley, chopped

Directions:

- ❖ In a heavy-bottomed pot, heat the olive over medium-high heat. Now, sauté the onion, carrot, parsnip, celery and yellow squash for about 3 minutes or until the vegetables are just tender.
- ❖ Add in the garlic and continue to sauté for 1 minute or until aromatic.
- ❖ Then, stir in the vegetable broth, tomatoes, quinoa, salt, pepper and bay laurel; bring to a boil. Immediately reduce the heat to a simmer and let it cook for 13 minutes.
- ❖ Fold in the Swiss chard; continue to simmer until the chard wilts.
- ❖ Ladle into individual bowls and serve garnished with the fresh parsley. Enjoy

162)   GREEN LENTIL SALAD

Preparation Time: 20 minutes + chilling time

Servings: 5

Ingredients:

- ✓ 1 ½ cups green lentils, rinsed
- ✓ 2 cups arugula
- ✓ 2 cups Romaine lettuce, torn into pieces
- ✓ 1 cup baby spinach
- ✓ 1/4 cup fresh basil, chopped
- ✓ 1/2 cup shallots, chopped
- ✓ 2 garlic cloves, finely chopped
- ✓ 1/4 cup oil-packed sun-dried tomatoes, rinsed and chopped
- ✓ 5 tbsp extra-virgin olive oil
- ✓ 3 tbsp fresh lemon juice
- ✓ Sea salt and ground black pepper, to taste

Directions:

- ❖ In a large-sized saucepan, bring 4 ½ cups of the water and red lentils to a boil.
- ❖ Immediately turn the heat to a simmer and continue to cook your lentils for a further 15 to 17 minutes or until they've softened but not mushy. Drain and let it cool completely.
- ❖ Transfer the lentils to a salad bowl; toss the lentils with the remaining ingredients until well combined.
- ❖ Serve chilled or at room temperature. Enjoy

163)   CHICKPEA, ACORN SQUASH, AND COUSCOUS SOUP

Preparation Time: 20 minutes

Servings: 4

Ingredients:

- ✓ 2 tbsp olive oil
- ✓ 1 shallot, chopped
- ✓ 1 carrot, trimmed and chopped
- ✓ 2 cups acorn squash, chopped
- ✓ 1 stalk celery, chopped
- ✓ 1 tsp garlic, finely chopped
- ✓ 1 tsp dried rosemary, chopped
- ✓ 1 tsp dried thyme, chopped
- ✓ 2 cups cream of onion soup
- ✓ 2 cups water
- ✓ 1 cup dry couscous
- ✓ Sea salt and ground black pepper, to taste
- ✓ 1/2 tsp red pepper flakes
- ✓ 6 ounces canned chickpeas, drained
- ✓ 2 tbsp fresh lemon juice

Directions:

- ❖ In a heavy-bottomed pot, heat the olive over medium-high heat. Now, sauté the shallot, carrot, acorn squash and celery for about 3 minutes or until the vegetables are just tender.
- ❖ Add in the garlic, rosemary and thyme and continue to sauté for 1 minute or until aromatic.
- ❖ Then, stir in the soup, water, couscous, salt, black pepper and red pepper flakes; bring to a boil. Immediately reduce the heat to a simmer and let it cook for 12 minutes.
- ❖ Fold in the canned chickpeas; continue to simmer until heated through or about 5 minutes more.
- ❖ Ladle into individual bowls and drizzle with the lemon juice over the top. Enjoy

164) GARLIC CROSTINI WITH CABBAGE SOUP

Preparation Time: 1 hour

Servings: 4

Ingredients:

- ✓ Soup:
- ✓ 2 tbsp olive oil
- ✓ 1 medium leek, chopped
- ✓ 1 cup turnip, chopped
- ✓ 1 parsnip, chopped
- ✓ 1 carrot, chopped
- ✓ 2 cups cabbage, shredded
- ✓ 2 garlic cloves, finely chopped
- ✓ 4 cups vegetable broth
- ✓ 2 bay leaves
- ✓ Sea salt and ground black pepper, to taste
- ✓ 1/4 tsp cumin seeds
- ✓ 1/2 tsp mustard seeds
- ✓ 1 tsp dried basil
- ✓ 2 tomatoes, pureed
- ✓ Crostini:
- ✓ 8 slices of baguette
- ✓ 2 heads garlic
- ✓ 4 tbsp extra-virgin olive oil

Directions:

- ❖ In a soup pot, heat 2 tbsp of the olive over medium-high heat. Now, sauté the leek, turnip, parsnip and carrot for about 4 minutes or until the vegetables are crisp-tender.
- ❖ Add in the garlic and cabbage and continue to sauté for 1 minute or until aromatic.
- ❖ Then, stir in the vegetable broth, bay leaves, salt, black pepper, cumin seeds, mustard seeds, dried basil and pureed tomatoes; bring to a boil. Immediately reduce the heat to a simmer and let it cook for about 20 minutes.
- ❖ Meanwhile, preheat your oven to 375 degrees F. Now, roast the garlic and baguette slices for about 15 minutes. Remove the crostini from the oven.
- ❖ Continue baking the garlic for 45 minutes more or until very tender. Allow the garlic to cool.
- ❖ Now, cut each head of the garlic using a sharp serrated knife in order to separate all the cloves.
- ❖ Squeeze the roasted garlic cloves out of their skins. Mash the garlic pulp with 4 tbsp of the extra-virgin olive oil.
- ❖ Spread the roasted garlic mixture evenly on the tops of the crostini. Serve with the warm soup. Enjoy

165) GREEN BEAN SOUP CREAM

Preparation Time: 35 minutes

Servings: 4

Ingredients:

- ✓ 1 tbsp sesame oil
- ✓ 1 onion, chopped
- ✓ 1 green pepper, seeded and chopped
- ✓ 2 russet potatoes, peeled and diced
- ✓ 2 garlic cloves, chopped
- ✓ 4 cups vegetable broth
- ✓ 1 pound green beans, trimmed
- ✓ Sea salt and ground black pepper, to season
- ✓ 1 cup full-fat coconut milk

Directions:

- ❖ In a heavy-bottomed pot, heat the sesame over medium-high heat. Now, sauté the onion, peppers and potatoes for about 5 minutes, stirring periodically. Add in the garlic and continue sautéing for 1 minute or until fragrant.
- ❖ Then, stir in the vegetable broth, green beans, salt and black pepper; bring to a boil. Immediately reduce the heat to a simmer and let it cook for 20 minutes.
- ❖ Puree the green bean mixture using an immersion blender until creamy and uniform.
- ❖ Return the pureed mixture to the pot. Fold in the coconut milk and continue to simmer until heated through or about 5 minutes longer.
- ❖ Ladle into individual bowls and serve hot. Enjoy

166) FRENCH TRADITIONAL ONION SOUP

Preparation Time: 1 hour 30 minutes

Servings: 4

Ingredients:

- ✓ 2 tbsp olive oil
- ✓ 2 large yellow onions, thinly sliced
- ✓ 2 thyme sprigs, chopped
- ✓ 2 rosemary sprigs, chopped
- ✓ 2 tsp balsamic vinegar
- ✓ 4 cups vegetable stock
- ✓ Sea salt and ground black pepper, to taste

Directions:

- ❖ In a or Dutch oven, heat the olive oil over a moderate heat. Now, cook the onions with thyme, rosemary and 1 tsp of the sea salt for about 2 minutes.
- ❖ Now, turn the heat to medium-low and continue cooking until the onions caramelize or about 50 minutes.
- ❖ Add in the balsamic vinegar and continue to cook for a further 15 more. Add in the stock, salt and black pepper and continue simmering for 20 to 25 minutes.
- ❖ Serve with toasted bread and enjoy

167) ROASTED CARROT SOUP

Preparation Time: 50 minutes

Servings: 4

Ingredients:

- ✓ 1 ½ pounds carrots
- ✓ 4 tbsp olive oil
- ✓ 1 yellow onion, chopped
- ✓ 2 cloves garlic, minced
- ✓ 1/3 tsp ground cumin
- ✓ Sea salt and white pepper, to taste
- ✓ 1/2 tsp turmeric powder
- ✓ 4 cups vegetable stock
- ✓ 2 tsp lemon juice
- ✓ 2 tbsp fresh cilantro, roughly chopped

Directions:

- ❖ Start by preheating your oven to 400 degrees F. Place the carrots on a large parchment-lined baking sheet; toss the carrots with 2 tbsp of the olive oil.
- ❖ Roast the carrots for about 35 minutes or until they've softened.
- ❖ In a heavy-bottomed pot, heat the remaining 2 tbsp of the olive-oil. Now, sauté the onion and garlic for about 3 minutes or until aromatic.
- ❖ Add in the cumin, salt, pepper, turmeric, vegetable stock and roasted carrots. Continue to simmer for 12 minutes more.
- ❖ Puree your soup with an immersion blender. Drizzle lemon juice over your soup and serve garnished with fresh cilantro leaves. Enjoy

168) ITALIAN PENNE PASTA SALAD

Preparation Time: 15 minutes + chilling time

Servings: 3

Ingredients:

- ✓ 9 ounces penne pasta
- ✓ 9 ounces canned Cannellini bean, drained
- ✓ 1 small onion, thinly sliced
- ✓ 1/3 cup Niçoise olives, pitted and sliced
- ✓ 2 Italian peppers, sliced
- ✓ 1 cup cherry tomatoes, halved
- ✓ 3 cups arugula

- ✓ Dressing:
- ✓ 3 tbsp extra-virgin olive oil
- ✓ 1 tsp lemon zest
- ✓ 1 tsp garlic, minced
- ✓ 3 tbsp balsamic vinegar
- ✓ 1 tsp Italian herb mix
- ✓ Sea salt and ground black pepper, to taste

Directions:

- ❖ Cook the penne pasta according to the package directions. Drain and rinse the pasta. Let it cool completely and then, transfer it to a salad bowl.
- ❖ Then, add the beans, onion, olives, peppers, tomatoes and arugula to the salad bowl.
- ❖ Mix all the dressing ingredients until everything is well incorporated. Dress your salad and serve well

169) CHANA CHAAT INDIAN SALAD

Preparation Time: 45 minutes + chilling time

Servings: 4

Ingredients:

- ✓ 1 pound dry chickpeas, soaked overnight
- ✓ 2 San Marzano tomatoes, diced
- ✓ 1 Persian cucumber, sliced
- ✓ 1 onion, chopped
- ✓ 1 bell pepper, seeded and thinly sliced
- ✓ 1 green chili, seeded and thinly sliced
- ✓ 2 handfuls baby spinach
- ✓ 1/2 tsp Kashmiri chili powder

- ✓ 4 curry leaves, chopped
- ✓ 1 tbsp chaat masala
- ✓ 2 tbsp fresh lemon juice, or to taste
- ✓ 4 tbsp olive oil
- ✓ 1 tsp agave syrup
- ✓ 1/2 tsp mustard seeds
- ✓ 1/2 tsp coriander seeds
- ✓ 2 tbsp sesame seeds, lightly toasted
- ✓ 2 tbsp fresh cilantro, roughly chopped

Directions:

- ❖ Drain the chickpeas and transfer them to a large saucepan. Cover the chickpeas with water by 2 inches and bring it to a boil.
- ❖ Immediately turn the heat to a simmer and continue to cook for approximately 40 minutes.
- ❖ Toss the chickpeas with the tomatoes, cucumber, onion, peppers, spinach, chili powder, curry leaves and chaat masala.
- ❖ In a small mixing dish, thoroughly combine the lemon juice, olive oil, agave syrup, mustard seeds and coriander seeds.
- ❖ Garnish with sesame seeds and fresh cilantro. Enjoy

170) **TEMPEH AND NOODLE SALAD THAI-STYLE**

Preparation Time: 45 minutes   **Servings: 3**

Ingredients:

- ✓ 6 ounces tempeh
- ✓ 4 tbsp rice vinegar
- ✓ 4 tbsp soy sauce
- ✓ 2 garlic cloves, minced
- ✓ 1 small-sized lime, freshly juiced
- ✓ 5 ounces rice noodles

- ✓ 1 carrot, julienned
- ✓ 1 shallot, chopped
- ✓ 3 handfuls Chinese cabbage, thinly sliced
- ✓ 3 handfuls kale, torn into pieces
- ✓ 1 bell pepper, seeded and thinly sliced
- ✓ 1 bird's eye chili, minced
- ✓ 1/4 cup peanut butter
- ✓ 2 tbsp agave syrup

Directions:

- ❖ Place the tempeh, 2 tbsp of the rice vinegar, soy sauce, garlic and lime juice in a ceramic dish; let it marinate for about 40 minutes.
- ❖ Meanwhile, cook the rice noodles according to the package directions. Drain your noodles and transfer them to a salad bowl.
- ❖ Add the carrot, shallot, cabbage, kale and peppers to the salad bowl. Add in the peanut butter, the remaining 2 tbsp of the rice vinegar and agave syrup and toss to combine well.
- ❖ Top with the marinated tempeh and serve immediately. Enjoy

171) **TYPICAL CREAM OF BROCCOLI SOUP**

Preparation Time: 35 minutes   **Servings: 4**

Ingredients:

- ✓ 2 tbsp olive oil
- ✓ 1 pound broccoli florets
- ✓ 1 onion, chopped
- ✓ 1 celery rib, chopped
- ✓ 1 parsnip, chopped
- ✓ 1 tsp garlic, chopped
- ✓ 3 cups vegetable broth

- ✓ 1/2 tsp dried dill
- ✓ 1/2 tsp dried oregano
- ✓ Sea salt and ground black pepper, to taste
- ✓ 2 tbsp flaxseed meal
- ✓ 1 cup full-fat coconut milk

Directions:

- ❖ In a heavy-bottomed pot, heat the olive oil over medium-high heat. Now, sauté the broccoli onion, celery and parsnip for about 5 minutes, stirring periodically.
- ❖ Add in the garlic and continue sautéing for 1 minute or until fragrant.
- ❖ Then, stir in the vegetable broth, dill, oregano, salt and black pepper; bring to a boil. Immediately reduce the heat to a simmer and let it cook for about 20 minutes.
- ❖ Puree the soup using an immersion blender until creamy and uniform.
- ❖ Return the pureed mixture to the pot. Fold in the flaxseed meal and coconut milk; continue to simmer until heated through or about 5 minutes.
- ❖ Ladle into four serving bowls and enjoy

172) RAISIN MOROCCAN LENTIL SALAD

Preparation Time: 20 minutes + chilling time

Servings: 4

Ingredients:

- ✓ 1 cup red lentils, rinsed
- ✓ 1 large carrot, julienned
- ✓ 1 Persian cucumber, thinly sliced
- ✓ 1 sweet onion, chopped
- ✓ 1/2 cup golden raisins
- ✓ 1/4 cup fresh mint, snipped
- ✓ 1/4 cup fresh basil, snipped
- ✓ 1/4 cup extra-virgin olive oil
- ✓ 1/4 cup lemon juice, freshly squeezed
- ✓ 1 tsp grated lemon peel
- ✓ 1/2 tsp fresh ginger root, peeled and minced
- ✓ 1/2 tsp granulated garlic
- ✓ 1 tsp ground allspice
- ✓ Sea salt and ground black pepper, to taste

Directions:

- ❖ In a large-sized saucepan, bring 3 cups of the water and 1 cup of the lentils to a boil.
- ❖ Immediately turn the heat to a simmer and continue to cook your lentils for a further 15 to 17 minutes or until they've softened but are not mushy yet. Drain and let it cool completely.
- ❖ Transfer the lentils to a salad bowl; add in the carrot, cucumber and sweet onion. Then, add the raisins, mint and basil to your salad.
- ❖ In a small mixing dish, whisk the olive oil, lemon juice, lemon peel, ginger, granulated garlic, allspice, salt and black pepper.
- ❖ Dress your salad and serve well-chilled. Enjoy

173) CHICKPEA AND ASPARAGUS SALAD

Preparation Time: 10 minutes + chilling time

Servings: 5

Ingredients:

- ✓ 1 ¼ pounds asparagus, trimmed and cut into bite-sized pieces
- ✓ 5 ounces canned chickpeas, drained and rinsed
- ✓ 1 chipotle pepper, seeded and chopped
- ✓ 1 Italian pepper, seeded and chopped
- ✓ 1/4 cup fresh basil leaves, chopped
- ✓ 1/4 cup fresh parsley leaves, chopped
- ✓ 2 tbsp fresh mint leaves
- ✓ 2 tbsp fresh chives, chopped
- ✓ 1 tsp garlic, minced
- ✓ 1/4 cup extra-virgin olive oil
- ✓ 1 tbsp balsamic vinegar
- ✓ 1 tbsp fresh lime juice
- ✓ 2 tbsp soy sauce
- ✓ 1/4 tsp ground allspice
- ✓ 1/4 tsp ground cumin
- ✓ Sea salt and freshly cracked peppercorns, to taste

Directions:

- ❖ Bring a large pot of salted water with the asparagus to a boil; let it cook for 2 minutes; drain and rinse.
- ❖ Transfer the asparagus to a salad bowl.
- ❖ Toss the asparagus with the chickpeas, peppers, herbs, garlic, olive oil, vinegar, lime juice, soy sauce and spices.
- ❖ Toss to combine and serve immediately. Enjoy

174)   QUINOA AND AVOCADO SALAD

Preparation Time: 15 minutes +

chilling time

Servings: 4

Ingredients:

- ✓ 1 cup quinoa, rinsed
- ✓ 1 onion, chopped
- ✓ 1 tomato, diced
- ✓ 2 roasted peppers, cut into strips
- ✓ 2 tbsp parsley, chopped
- ✓ 2 tbsp basil, chopped
- ✓ 1/4 cup extra-virgin olive oil
- ✓ 2 tbsp red wine vinegar
- ✓ 2 tbsp lemon juice
- ✓ 1/4 tsp cayenne pepper
- ✓ Sea salt and freshly ground black pepper, to season
- ✓ 1 avocado, peeled, pitted and sliced
- ✓ 1 tbsp sesame seeds, toasted

Directions:

- ❖ Place the water and quinoa in a saucepan and bring it to a rolling boil. Immediately turn the heat to a simmer.
- ❖ Let it simmer for about 13 minutes until the quinoa has absorbed all of the water; fluff the quinoa with a fork and let it cool completely. Then, transfer the quinoa to a salad bowl.
- ❖ Add the onion, tomato, roasted peppers, parsley and basil to the salad bowl. In another small bowl, whisk the olive oil, vinegar, lemon juice, cayenne pepper, salt and black pepper.
- ❖ Dress your salad and toss to combine well. Top with avocado slices and garnish with toasted sesame seeds.
- ❖ Enjoy

175)   TABBOULEH SALAD WITH TOFU

Preparation Time: 20 minutes +

chilling time

Servings: 4

Ingredients:

- ✓ 1 cup bulgur wheat
- ✓ 2 San Marzano tomatoes, sliced
- ✓ 1 Persian cucumber, thinly sliced
- ✓ 2 tbsp basil, chopped
- ✓ 2 tbsp parsley, chopped
- ✓ 4 scallions, chopped
- ✓ 2 cups arugula
- ✓ 2 cups baby spinach, torn into pieces
- ✓ 4 tbsp tahini
- ✓ 4 tbsp lemon juice
- ✓ 1 tbsp soy sauce
- ✓ 1 tsp fresh garlic, pressed
- ✓ Sea salt and ground black pepper, to taste
- ✓ 12 ounces smoked tofu, cubed

Directions:

- ❖ In a saucepan, bring 2 cups of water and the bulgur to a boil. Immediately turn the heat to a simmer and let it cook for about 20 minutes or until the bulgur is tender and the water is almost absorbed. Fluff with a fork and spread on a large tray to let cool.
- ❖ Place the bulgur in a salad bowl followed by the tomatoes, cucumber, basil, parsley, scallions, arugula and spinach.
- ❖ In a small mixing dish, whisk the tahini, lemon juice, soy sauce, garlic, salt and black pepper. Dress the salad and toss to combine.
- ❖ Top your salad with the smoked tofu and serve at room temperature. Enjoy

176)   GREEN PASTA SALAD

Preparation Time: 10 minutes +

chilling time

Servings: 4

Ingredients:

- ✓ 12 ounces rotini pasta
- ✓ 1 small onion, thinly sliced
- ✓ 1 cup cherry tomatoes, halved
- ✓ 1 bell pepper, chopped
- ✓ 1 jalapeno pepper, chopped
- ✓ 1 tbsp capers, drained
- ✓ 2 cups Iceberg lettuce, torn into pieces
- ✓ 2 tbsp fresh parsley, chopped
- ✓ 2 tbsp fresh cilantro, chopped
- ✓ 2 tbsp fresh basil, chopped
- ✓ 1/4 cup olive oil
- ✓ 2 tbsp apple cider vinegar
- ✓ 1 tsp garlic, pressed
- ✓ Kosher salt and ground black pepper, to taste
- ✓ 2 tbsp nutritional yeast
- ✓ 2 tbsp pine nuts, toasted and chopped

Directions:

- ❖ Cook the pasta according to the package directions. Drain and rinse the pasta. Let it cool completely and then, transfer it to a salad bowl.
- ❖ Then, add in the onion, tomatoes, peppers, capers, lettuce, parsley, cilantro and basil to the salad bowl.
- ❖ Whisk the olive oil, vinegar, garlic, salt, black pepper and nutritional yeast. Dress your salad and top with toasted pine nuts. Enjoy

177)   ORIGINAL UKRAINIAN BORSCHT

Preparation Time: 40 minutes

Servings: 4

Ingredients:

- 2 tbsp sesame oil
- 1 red onion, chopped
- 2 carrots, trimmed and sliced
- 2 large beets, peeled and sliced
- 2 large potatoes, peeled and diced
- 4 cups vegetable stock
- 2 garlic cloves, minced
- 1/2 tsp caraway seeds
- 1/2 tsp celery seeds
- 1/2 tsp fennel seeds
- 1 pound red cabbage, shredded
- 1/2 tsp mixed peppercorns, freshly cracked
- Kosher salt, to taste
- 2 bay leaves
- 2 tbsp wine vinegar

Directions:

- In a Dutch oven, heat the sesame oil over a moderate flame. Once hot, sauté the onions until tender and translucent, about 6 minutes.
- Add in the carrots, beets and potatoes and continue to sauté an additional 10 minutes, adding the vegetable stock periodically.
- Next, stir in the garlic, caraway seeds, celery seeds, fennel seeds and continue sautéing for another 30 seconds.
- Add in the cabbage, mixed peppercorns, salt and bay leaves. Add in the remaining stock and bring to boil.
- Immediately turn the heat to a simmer and continue to cook for 20 to 23 minutes longer until the vegetables have softened.
- Ladle into individual bowls and drizzle wine vinegar over it. Serve and enjoy

178)   LENTIL BELUGA SALAD

Preparation Time: 20 minutes + chilling time

Servings: 4

Ingredients:

- 1 cup Beluga lentils, rinsed
- 1 Persian cucumber, sliced
- 1 large-sized tomatoes, sliced
- 1 red onion, chopped
- 1 bell pepper, sliced
- 1/4 cup fresh basil, chopped
- 1/4 cup fresh Italian parsley, chopped
- 2 ounces green olives, pitted and sliced
- 1/4 cup olive oil
- 4 tbsp lemon juice
- 1 tsp deli mustard
- 1/2 tsp garlic, minced
- 1/2 tsp red pepper flakes, crushed
- Sea salt and ground black pepper, to taste

Directions:

- In a large-sized saucepan, bring 3 cups of the water and 1 cup of the lentils to a boil.
- Immediately turn the heat to a simmer and continue to cook your lentils for a further 15 to 17 minutes or until they've softened but not mushy. Drain and let it cool completely.
- Transfer the lentils to a salad bowl; add in the cucumber, tomatoes, onion, pepper, basil, parsley and olives.
- In a small mixing dish, whisk the olive oil, lemon juice, mustard, garlic, red pepper, salt and black pepper.
- Dress the salad, toss to combine and serve well-chilled. Enjoy

179)   INDIAN NAAN SALAD

Preparation Time: 10 minutes

Servings: 3

Ingredients:

- ✓ 3 tbsp sesame oil
- ✓ 1 tsp ginger, peeled and minced
- ✓ 1/2 tsp cumin seeds
- ✓ 1/2 tsp mustard seeds
- ✓ 1/2 tsp mixed peppercorns
- ✓ 1 tbsp curry leaves
- ✓ 3 naan breads, broken into bite-sized pieces
- ✓ 1 shallot, chopped
- ✓ 2 tomatoes, chopped
- ✓ Himalayan salt, to taste
- ✓ 1 tbsp soy sauce

Directions:

- ❖ Heat 2 tbsp of the sesame oil in a non-stick skillet over a moderately high heat.
- ❖ Sauté the ginger, cumin seeds, mustard seeds, mixed peppercorns and curry leaves for 1 minute or so, until fragrant.
- ❖ Stir in the naan breads and continue to cook, stirring periodically, until golden-brown and well coated with the spices.
- ❖ Place the shallot and tomatoes in a salad bowl; toss them with the salt, soy sauce and the remaining 1 tbsp of the sesame oil.
- ❖ Place the toasted naan on the top of your salad and serve at room temperature. Enjoy

180)   BROCCOLI GINGER SOUP

Preparation Time: 50 minutes

Servings: 4

Ingredients:

- ✓ 1 onion, chopped
- ✓ 1 tbsp minced peeled fresh ginger
- ✓ 2 tsp olive oil
- ✓ 2 carrots, chopped
- ✓ 1 head broccoli, chopped into florets
- ✓ 1 cup coconut milk
- ✓ 3 cups vegetable broth
- ✓ ½ tsp turmeric
- ✓ Salt and black pepper to taste

Directions:

- ❖ In a pot over medium heat, place the onion, ginger, and olive oil, cook for 4 minutes. Add in carrots, broccoli, broth, turmeric, pepper, and salt. Bring to a boil and cook for 15 minutes. Transfer the soup to a food processor and blend until smooth. Stir in coconut milk and serve warm

181)   NOODLE RICE SOUP WITH BEANS

Preparation Time: 10 minutes

Servings: 6

Ingredients:

- ✓ 2 carrots, chopped
- ✓ 2 celery stalks, chopped
- ✓ 6 cups vegetable broth
- ✓ 8 oz brown rice noodles
- ✓ 1 (15-oz) can pinto beans
- ✓ 1 tsp dried herbs

Directions:

- ❖ Place a pot over medium heat and add in the carrots, celery, and vegetable broth. Bring to a boil. Add in noodles, beans, dried herbs, salt, and pepper. Reduce the heat and simmer for 5 minutes. Serve

182) VEGETABLE AND RICE SOUP

Preparation Time: 40 minutes

Servings: 6

Ingredients:

- ✓ 3 tbsp olive oil
- ✓ 2 carrots, chopped
- ✓ 1 onion, chopped
- ✓ 1 celery stalk, chopped
- ✓ 2 garlic cloves, minced
- ✓ 2 cups chopped cabbage
- ✓ ½ red bell pepper, chopped
- ✓ 4 potatoes, unpeeled and quartered
- ✓ 6 cups vegetable broth
- ✓ ½ cup brown rice, rinsed
- ✓ ½ cup frozen green peas
- ✓ 2 tbsp chopped parsley

Directions:

- ❖ Heat the oil in a pot over medium heat. Place carrots, onion, celery, and garlic. Cook for 5 minutes. Add in cabbage, bell pepper, potatoes, and broth. Bring to a boil, then lower the heat and add the brown rice, salt, and pepper. Simmer uncovered for 25 minutes until vegetables are tender. Stir in peas and cook for 5 minutes. Top with parsley and serve warm

183) DAIKON AND SWEET POTATO SOUP

Preparation Time: 40 minutes

Servings: 6

Ingredients:

- ✓ 6 cups water
- ✓ 2 tsp olive oil
- ✓ 1 chopped onion
- ✓ 3 garlic cloves, minced
- ✓ 1 tbsp thyme
- ✓ 2 tsp paprika
- ✓ 2 cups peeled and chopped daikon
- ✓ 2 cups chopped sweet potatoes
- ✓ 2 cups peeled and chopped parsnips
- ✓ ½ tsp sea salt
- ✓ 1 cup fresh mint, chopped
- ✓ ½ avocado
- ✓ 2 tbsp balsamic vinegar
- ✓ 2 tbsp pumpkin seeds

Directions:

- ❖ Heat the oil in a pot and place onion and garlic. Sauté for 3 minutes. Add in thyme, paprika, daikon, sweet potato, parsnips, water, and salt. Bring to a boil and cook for 30 minutes. Remove the soup to a food processor and add in balsamic vinegar; purée until smooth. Top with mint and pumpkin seeds to serve

184) CHICKPEA AND VEGETABLE SOUP

Preparation Time: 35 minutes

Servings: 5

Ingredients:

- ✓ 2 tbsp olive oil
- ✓ 1 onion, chopped
- ✓ 1 carrot, chopped
- ✓ 1 celery stalk, chopped
- ✓ 2 tsp smoked paprika
- ✓ 1 tsp ground cumin
- ✓ 1 tsp za'atar spice
- ✓ ¼ tsp ground cayenne pepper
- ✓ 6 cups vegetable

Directions:

- ❖ Heat the oil in a pot over medium heat. Place onion, carrot, and celery and cook for 5 minutes. Add in eggplant, tomatoes, tomato paste, chickpeas, paprika, cumin, za´atar spice, and cayenne pepper. Stir in broth and salt. Bring to a

- ✓ 1 eggplant, chopped
- ✓ 1 (28-oz) can diced tomatoes
- ✓ 2 tbsp tomato paste
- ✓ 1 (15.5-oz) can chickpeas, drained

broth
- ✓ 4 oz whole-wheat vermicelli
- ✓ 2 tbsp minced cilantro

boil, then lower the heat and simmer for 15 minutes. Add in vermicelli and cook for another 5 minutes. Serve topped with cilantro

185) ITALIAN-STYLE BEAN SOUP

Preparation Time: 1 hour 25 minutes

Servings: 6

Ingredients:

- ✓ 3 tbsp olive oil
- ✓ 2 celery stalks, chopped
- ✓ 2 carrots, chopped
- ✓ 3 shallots, chopped
- ✓ 3 garlic cloves, minced
- ✓ ½ cup brown rice
- ✓ 6 cups vegetable broth
- ✓ 1 (14.5-oz) can diced tomatoes
- ✓ 2 bay leaves
- ✓ Salt and black pepper to taste
- ✓ 2 (15.5-oz) cans white beans
- ✓ ¼ cup chopped basil

Directions:

- ❖ Heat oil in a pot over medium heat. Place celery, carrots, shallots, and garlic and cook for 5 minutes. Add in brown rice, broth, tomatoes, bay leaves, salt, and pepper. Bring to a boil, then lower the heat and simmer uncovered for 20 minutes. Stir in beans and basil and cook for 5 minutes. Discard bay leaves and spoon into bowls. Sprinkle with basil and serve

186) BRUSSELS SPROUTS AND TOFU SOUP

Preparation Time: 40 minutes

Servings: 4

Ingredients:

- ✓ 7 oz firm tofu, cubed
- ✓ 2 tsp olive oil
- ✓ 1 cup sliced mushrooms
- ✓ 1 cup shredded Brussels sprouts
- ✓ 1 garlic clove, minced
- ✓ ½-inch piece fresh ginger, minced
- ✓ Salt to taste
- ✓ 2 tbsp apple cider vinegar
- ✓ 2 tbsp soy sauce
- ✓ 1 tsp pure date sugar
- ✓ ¼ tsp red pepper flakes
- ✓ 1 scallion, chopped

Directions:

- ❖ Heat the oil in a skillet over medium heat. Place mushrooms, Brussels sprouts, garlic, ginger, and salt. Sauté for 7-8 minutes until the veggies are soft. Pour in 4 cups of water, vinegar, soy sauce, sugar, pepper flakes, and tofu. Bring to a boil, then lower the heat and simmer for 5-10 minutes. Top with scallions and serve

187) WHITE BEAN ROSEMARY SOUP

Preparation Time: 30 minutes

Servings: 4

Ingredients:

- ✓ 2 tsp olive oil
- ✓ 1 carrot, chopped
- ✓ 1 onion, chopped
- ✓ 2 garlic cloves, minced
- ✓ 1 tbsp rosemary, chopped
- ✓ 2 tbsp apple cider vinegar
- ✓ 1 cup dried white beans
- ✓ ¼ tsp salt
- ✓ 2 tbsp nutritional yeast

Directions:

- ❖ Heat the oil in a pot over medium heat. Place carrots, onion, and garlic and cook for 5 minutes.
- ❖ Pour in vinegar to deglaze the pot. Stir in 5 cups water and beans and bring to a boil. Lower the heat and simmer for 45 minutes until the beans are soft. Add in salt and nutritional yeast and stir. Serve topped with chopped rosemary

188) MUSHROOM AND TOFU SOUP

Preparation Time: 20 minutes

Servings: 4

Ingredients:

- ✓ 4 cups water
- ✓ 2 tbsp soy sauce
- ✓ 4 white mushrooms, sliced
- ✓ ¼ cup chopped green onions
- ✓ 3 tbsp tahini
- ✓ 6 oz extra-firm tofu, diced

Directions:

- ❖ Pour the water and soy sauce into a pot and bring to a boil. Add in mushrooms and green onions. Lower the heat and simmer for 10 minutes. In a bowl, combine ½ cup of hot soup with tahini. Pour the mixture into the pot and simmer 2 minutes more, but not boil. Stir in tofu. Serve warm

189) AUTUMN ROOT VEGETABLE SOUP

Preparation Time: 40 minutes

Servings: 4

Ingredients:

- ✓ 4 tbsp avocado oil
- ✓ 1 large leek, sliced
- ✓ 2 carrots, diced
- ✓ 2 parsnips, diced
- ✓ 2 cups turnip, diced
- ✓ 2 celery stalks, diced
- ✓ 1 pound sweet potatoes, diced
- ✓ 1 tsp ginger-garlic paste
- ✓ 1 habanero pepper, seeded and chopped
- ✓ 1/2 tsp caraway seeds
- ✓ 1/2 tsp fennel seeds
- ✓ 2 bay leaves
- ✓ Sea salt and ground black pepper, to season
- ✓ 1 tsp cayenne pepper
- ✓ 4 cups vegetable broth
- ✓ 4 tbsp tahini

Directions:

- ❖ In a stockpot, heat the oil over medium-high heat. Now, sauté the leeks, carrots, parsnip, turnip, celery and sweet potatoes for about 5 minutes, stirring periodically.
- ❖ Add in the ginger-garlic paste and habanero peppers and continue sautéing for 1 minute or until fragrant.
- ❖ Then, stir in the caraway seeds, fennel seeds, bay leaves, salt, black pepper, cayenne pepper and vegetable broth; bring to a boil. Immediately turn the heat to a simmer and let it cook for approximately 25 minutes.
- ❖ Puree the soup using an immersion blender until creamy and uniform.
- ❖ Return the pureed mixture to the pot. Fold in the tahini and continue to simmer until heated through or about 5 minutes longer.
- ❖ Ladle into individual bowls and serve hot. Enjoy

190) GREEK SALAD

Preparation Time: 10 minutes

Servings: 2

Ingredients:

- ✓ ½ yellow bell pepper, cut into pieces
- ✓ 3 tomatoes cut into bite-size pieces
- ✓ ½ cucumber, cut into
- ✓ ½ cup tofu cheese, cut into squares
- ✓ 10 Kalamata olives, pitted
- ✓ ½ tbsp red wine vinegar
- ✓ 4 tbsp olive oil

Directions:

- ❖ Pour the bell pepper, tomatoes, cucumber, red onion, tofu cheese, and olives into a salad bowl. Drizzle the red wine vinegar and olive oil over the vegetables. Season with salt, black pepper, and oregano, and toss the salad with two spoons. Share

bite-size pieces

✓ ½ red onion, peeled and sliced

✓ 2 tsp dried oregano

the salad into two bowls and serve immediately

VEGETABLES AND SIDE DISHES

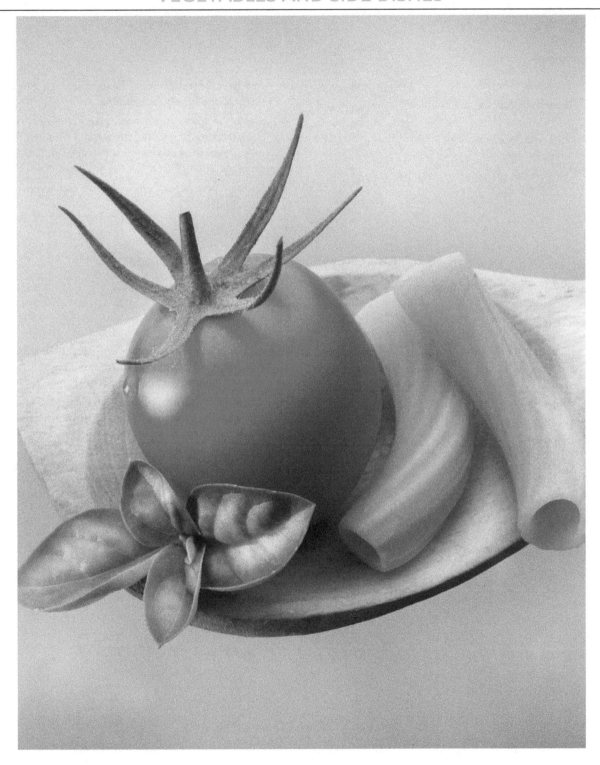

191) CHINESE CABBAGE STIR-FRY

Preparation Time: 10 minutes

Servings: 3

Ingredients:

- ✓ 3 tbsp sesame oil
- ✓ 1 pound Chinese cabbage, sliced
- ✓ 1/2 tsp Chinese five-spice powder
- ✓ Kosher salt, to taste
- ✓ 1/2 tsp Szechuan pepper
- ✓ 2 tbsp soy sauce
- ✓ 3 tbsp sesame seeds, lightly toasted

Directions:

- ❖ In a wok, heat the sesame oil until sizzling. Stir fry the cabbage for about 5 minutes.
- ❖ Stir in the spices and soy sauce and continue to cook, stirring frequently, for about 5 minutes more, until the cabbage is crisp-tender and aromatic.
- ❖ Sprinkle sesame seeds over the top and serve immediately

192) SAUTÉED CAULIFLOWER WITH SESAME SEEDS

Preparation Time: 15 minutes

Servings: 4

Ingredients:

- ✓ 1 cup vegetable broth
- ✓ 1 ½ pounds cauliflower florets
- ✓ 4 tbsp olive oil
- ✓ 2 scallion stalks, chopped
- ✓ 4 garlic cloves, minced
- ✓ Sea salt and freshly ground black pepper, to taste
- ✓ 2 tbsp sesame seeds, lightly toasted

Directions:

- ❖ In a large saucepan, bring the vegetable broth to a boil; then, add in the cauliflower and cook for about 6 minutes or until fork-tender; reserve.
- ❖ Then, heat the olive oil until sizzling; now, sauté the scallions and garlic for about 1 minute or until tender and aromatic.
- ❖ Add in the reserved cauliflower, followed by salt and black pepper; continue to simmer for about 5 minutes or until heated through
- ❖ Garnish with toasted sesame seeds and serve immediately. Enjoy

193)   SWEET MASHED CARROTS

Preparation Time: 25 minutes

Servings: 4

Ingredients:

- ✓ 1 ½ pounds carrots, trimmed
- ✓ 3 tbsp vegan butter
- ✓ 1 cup scallions, sliced
- ✓ 1 tbsp maple syrup
- ✓ 1/2 tsp garlic powder
- ✓ 1/2 tsp ground allspice
- ✓ Sea salt, to taste
- ✓ 1/2 cup soy sauce
- ✓ 2 tbsp fresh cilantro, chopped

Directions:

- ❖ Steam the carrots for about 15 minutes until they are very tender; drain well.
- ❖ In a sauté pan, melt the butter until sizzling. Now, turn the heat down to maintain an insistent sizzle.
- ❖ Now, cook the scallions until they've softened. Add in the maple syrup, garlic powder, ground allspice, salt and soy sauce for about 10 minutes or until they are caramelized.
- ❖ Add the caramelized scallions to your food processor; add in the carrots and puree the ingredients until everything is well blended.
- ❖ Serve garnished with the fresh cilantro. Enjoy

194)   SAUTÉED TURNIP GREENS

Preparation Time: 15 minutes

Servings: 4

Ingredients:

- ✓ 2 tbsp olive oil
- ✓ 1 onion, sliced
- ✓ 2 garlic cloves, sliced
- ✓ 1 ½ pounds turnip greens cleaned and chopped
- ✓ 1/4 cup vegetable broth
- ✓ 1/4 cup dry white wine
- ✓ 1/2 tsp dried oregano
- ✓ 1 tsp dried parsley flakes
- ✓ Kosher salt and ground black pepper, to taste

Directions:

- ❖ In a sauté pan, heat the olive oil over a moderately high heat.
- ❖ Now, sauté the onion for 3 to 4 minutes or until tender and translucent. Add in the garlic and continue to cook for 30 seconds more or until aromatic.
- ❖ Stir in the turnip greens, broth, wine, oregano and parsley; continue sautéing an additional 6 minutes or until they have wilted completely.
- ❖ Season with salt and black pepper to taste and serve warm. Enjoy

195) YUKON GOLD MASHED POTATOES

Preparation Time: 25 minutes

Servings: 5

Ingredients:

- ✓ 2 pounds Yukon Gold potatoes, peeled and diced
- ✓ 1 clove garlic, pressed
- ✓ Sea salt and red pepper flakes, to taste
- ✓ 3 tbsp vegan butter
- ✓ 1/2 cup soy milk
- ✓ 2 tbsp scallions, sliced

Directions:

- ❖ Cover the potatoes with an inch or two of cold water. Cook the potatoes in gently boiling water for about 20 minutes.
- ❖ Then, puree the potatoes, along with the garlic, salt, red pepper, butter and milk, to your desired consistency.
- ❖ Serve garnished with fresh scallions. Enjoy

196) AROMATIC SAUTÉED SWISS CHARD

Preparation Time: 15 minutes

Servings: 4

Ingredients:

- ✓ 2 tbsp vegan butter
- ✓ 1 onion, chopped
- ✓ 2 cloves garlic, sliced
- ✓ Sea salt and ground black pepper, to season
- ✓ 1 ½ pounds Swiss chard, torn into pieces, tough stalks removed
- ✓ 1 cup vegetable broth
- ✓ 1 bay leaf
- ✓ 1 thyme sprig
- ✓ 2 rosemary sprigs
- ✓ 1/2 tsp mustard seeds
- ✓ 1 tsp celery seeds

Directions:

- ❖ In a saucepan, melt the vegan butter over medium-high heat.
- ❖ Then, sauté the onion for about 3 minutes or until tender and translucent; sauté the garlic for about 1 minute until aromatic.
- ❖ Add in the remaining ingredients and turn the heat to a simmer; let it simmer, covered, for about 10 minutes or until everything is cooked through. Enjoy

197) CLASSIC SAUTÉED BELL PEPPERS

Preparation Time: 15 minutes

Servings: 2

Ingredients:

- ✓ 3 tbsp olive oil
- ✓ 4 bell peppers, seeded and slice into strips
- ✓ 2 cloves garlic, minced
- ✓ Salt and freshly ground black pepper, to taste
- ✓ 1 tsp cayenne pepper
- ✓ 4 tbsp dry white wine
- ✓ 2 tbsp fresh cilantro, roughly chopped

Directions:

- ❖ In a saucepan, heat the oil over medium-high heat.
- ❖ Once hot, sauté the peppers for about 4 minutes or until tender and fragrant. Then, sauté the garlic for about 1 minute until aromatic.
- ❖ Add in the salt, black pepper and cayenne pepper; continue to sauté, adding the wine, for about 6 minutes more until tender and cooked through.
- ❖ Taste and adjust the seasonings. Top with fresh cilantro and serve. Enjoy

198) MASHED ROOT VEGETABLES

Preparation Time: 25 minutes

Servings: 5

Ingredients:

- ✓ 1 pound russet potatoes, peeled and cut into chunks
- ✓ 1/2 pound parsnips, trimmed and diced
- ✓ 1/2 pound carrots, trimmed and diced
- ✓ 4 tbsp vegan butter
- ✓ 1 tsp dried oregano
- ✓ 1/2 tsp dried dill weed
- ✓ 1/2 tsp dried marjoram
- ✓ 1 tsp dried basil

Directions:

- ❖ Cover the vegetables with the water by 1 inch. Bring to a boil and cook for about 25 minutes until they've softened; drain.
- ❖ Mash the vegetables with the remaining ingredients, adding cooking liquid, as needed.
- ❖ Serve warm and enjoy

199) ROASTED BUTTERNUT SQUASH

Preparation Time: 25 minutes

Servings: 4

Ingredients:

- ✓ 4 tbsp olive oil
- ✓ 1/2 tsp ground cumin
- ✓ 1/2 tsp ground allspice
- ✓ 1 ½ pounds butternut squash, peeled, seeded and diced
- ✓ 1/4 cup dry white wine
- ✓ 2 tbsp dark soy sauce
- ✓ 1 tsp mustard seeds
- ✓ 1 tsp paprika
- ✓ Sea salt and ground black pepper, to taste

Directions:

- ❖ Start by preheating your oven to 420 degrees F. Toss the squash with the remaining ingredients.
- ❖ Roast the butternut squash for about 25 minutes or until tender and caramelized.
- ❖ Serve warm and enjoy

200) SAUTÉED CREMINI MUSHROOMS

Preparation Time: 10 minutes

Servings: 4

Ingredients:

- ✓ 4 tbsp olive oil
- ✓ 4 tbsp shallots, chopped
- ✓ 2 cloves garlic, minced
- ✓ 1 ½ pounds Cremini mushrooms, sliced
- ✓ 1/4 cup dry white wine
- ✓ Sea salt and ground black pepper, to taste

Directions:

- ❖ In a sauté pan, heat the olive oil over a moderately high heat.
- ❖ Now, sauté the shallot for 3 to 4 minutes or until tender and translucent. Add in the garlic and continue to cook for 30 seconds more or until aromatic.
- ❖ Stir in the Cremini mushrooms, wine, salt and black pepper; continue sautéing an additional 6 minutes, until your mushrooms are lightly browned.
- ❖ Enjoy

201) ROASTED ASPARAGUS WITH SESAME SEEDS

Preparation Time: 25 minutes

Servings: 4

Ingredients:

- ✓ 1 ½ pounds asparagus, trimmed
- ✓ 4 tbsp extra-virgin olive oil
- ✓ Sea salt and ground black pepper, to taste
- ✓ 1/2 tsp dried oregano
- ✓ 1/2 tsp dried basil
- ✓ 1 tsp red pepper flakes, crushed
- ✓ 4 tbsp sesame seeds
- ✓ 2 tbsp fresh chives, roughly chopped

Directions:

- ❖ Start by preheating the oven to 400 degrees F. Then, line a baking sheet with parchment paper.
- ❖ Toss the asparagus with the olive oil, salt, black pepper, oregano, basil and red pepper flakes. Now, arrange your asparagus in a single layer on the prepared baking sheet.
- ❖ Roast your asparagus for approximately 20 minutes.
- ❖ Sprinkle sesame seeds over your asparagus and continue to bake an additional 5 minutes or until the asparagus spears are crisp-tender and the sesame seeds are lightly toasted.
- ❖ Garnish with fresh chives and serve warm. Enjoy

202) GREEK-STYLE EGGPLANT SKILLET

Preparation Time: 15 minutes

Servings: 4

Ingredients:

- ✓ 4 tbsp olive oil
- ✓ 1 ½ pounds eggplant, peeled and sliced
- ✓ 1 tsp garlic, minced
- ✓ 1 tomato, crushed
- ✓ Sea salt and ground black pepper, to taste
- ✓ 1 tsp cayenne pepper
- ✓ 1/2 tsp dried oregano
- ✓ 1/4 tsp ground bay leaf
- ✓ 2 ounces Kalamata olives, pitted and sliced

Directions:

- ❖ Heat the oil in a sauté pan over medium-high flame.
- ❖ Then, sauté the eggplant for about 9 minutes or until just tender.
- ❖ Add in the remaining ingredients, cover and continue to cook for 2 to 3 minutes more or until thoroughly cooked. Serve warm

203) CAULIFLOWER RICE

Preparation Time: 10 minutes

Servings: 5

Ingredients:

- ✓ 2 medium heads cauliflower, stems and leaves removed
- ✓ 4 tbsp extra-virgin olive oil
- ✓ 4 garlic cloves, pressed
- ✓ 1/2 tsp red pepper flakes, crushed
- ✓ Sea salt and ground black pepper, to taste
- ✓ 1/4 cup flat-leaf parsley, roughly chopped

Directions:

- ❖ Pulse the cauliflower in a food processor with the S-blade until they're broken into "rice".
- ❖ Heat the olive oil in a saucepan over medium-high heat. Once hot, cook the garlic until fragrant or about 1 minute.
- ❖ Add in the cauliflower rice, red pepper, salt and black pepper and continue sautéing for a further 7 to 8 minutes.
- ❖ Taste, adjust the seasonings and garnish with fresh parsley. Enjoy

204) GARLICKY KALE

Preparation Time: 10 minutes

Servings: 4

Ingredients:

- ✓ 4 tbsp olive oil
- ✓ 4 cloves garlic, chopped
- ✓ 1 ½ pounds fresh kale, tough stems and ribs removed, torn into pieces
- ✓ 1 cup vegetable broth
- ✓ 1/2 tsp cumin seeds
- ✓ 1/2 tsp dried oregano
- ✓ 1/2 tsp paprika
- ✓ 1 tsp onion powder
- ✓ Sea salt and ground black pepper, to taste

Directions:

- ❖ In a saucepan, heat the olive oil over a moderately high heat. Now, sauté the garlic for about 1 minute or until aromatic.
- ❖ Add in the kale in batches, gradually adding the vegetable broth; stir to promote even cooking.
- ❖ Turn the heat to a simmer, add in the spices and let it cook for 5 to 6 minutes, until the kale leaves wilt.
- ❖ Serve warm and enjoy

205) ARTICHOKES BRAISED IN LEMON AND OLIVE OIL

Preparation Time: 35 minutes   **Servings: 4**

Ingredients:

- ✓ 1 ½ cups water
- ✓ 2 lemons, freshly squeezed
- ✓ 2 pounds artichokes, trimmed, tough outer leaves and chokes removed
- ✓ 1 handful fresh Italian parsley
- ✓ 2 thyme sprigs
- ✓ 2 rosemary sprigs
- ✓ 2 bay leaves
- ✓ 2 garlic cloves, chopped
- ✓ 1/3 cup olive oil
- ✓ Sea salt and ground black pepper, to taste
- ✓ 1/2 tsp red pepper flakes

Directions:

- ❖ Fill a bowl with water and add in the lemon juice. Place the cleaned artichokes in the bowl, keeping them completely submerged.
- ❖ In another small bowl, thoroughly combine the herbs and garlic. Rub your artichokes with the herb mixture.
- ❖ Pour the lemon water and olive oil in a saucepan; add the artichokes to the saucepan. Turn the heat to a simmer and continue to cook, covered, for about 30 minutes until the artichokes are crisp-tender.
- ❖ To serve, drizzle the artichokes with cooking juices, season them with the salt, black pepper and red pepper flakes. Enjoy

206) ROSEMARY AND GARLIC ROASTED CARROTS

Preparation Time: 25 minutes   **Servings: 4**

Ingredients:

- ✓ 2 pounds carrots, trimmed and halved lengthwise
- ✓ 4 tbsp olive oil
- ✓ 2 tbsp champagne vinegar
- ✓ 4 cloves garlic, minced
- ✓ 2 sprigs rosemary, chopped
- ✓ Sea salt and ground black pepper, to taste
- ✓ 4 tbsp pine nuts, chopped

Directions:

- ❖ Begin by preheating your oven to 400 degrees F.
- ❖ Toss the carrots with the olive oil, vinegar, garlic, rosemary, salt and black pepper. Arrange them in a single layer on a parchment-lined roasting sheet.
- ❖ Roast the carrots in the preheated oven for about 20 minutes, until fork-tender.
- ❖ Garnish the carrots with the pine nuts and serve immediately. Enjoy

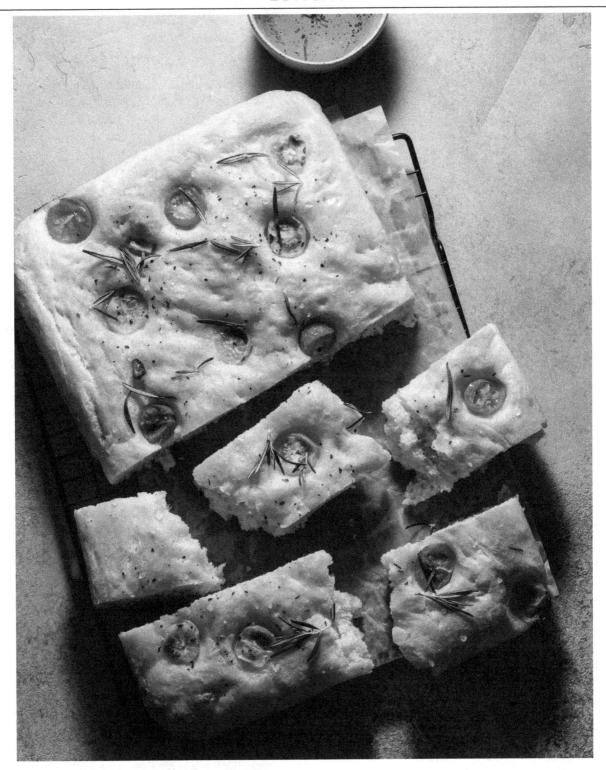

207) MILLET PORRIDGE WITH SULTANAS

Preparation Time: 25 minutes

Servings: 3

Ingredients:

- ✓ 1 cup water
- ✓ 1 cup coconut milk
- ✓ 1 cup millet, rinsed
- ✓ 1/4 tsp grated nutmeg
- ✓ 1⁄4 tsp ground cinnamon
- ✓ 1 tsp vanilla paste
- ✓ 1/4 tsp kosher salt
- ✓ 2 tbsp agave syrup
- ✓ 4 tbsp sultana raisins

Directions:

- ❖ Place the water, milk, millet, nutmeg, cinnamon, vanilla and salt in a saucepan; bring to a boil.
- ❖ Turn the heat to a simmer and let it cook for about 20 minutes; fluff the millet with a fork and spoon into individual bowls.
- ❖ Serve with agave syrup and sultanas. Enjoy

208) QUINOA PORRIDGE WITH DRIED FIGS

Preparation Time: 25 minutes

Servings: 3

Ingredients:

- ✓ 1 cup white quinoa, rinsed
- ✓ 2 cups almond milk
- ✓ 4 tbsp brown sugar
- ✓ A pinch of salt
- ✓ 1/4 tsp grated nutmeg
- ✓ 1/2 tsp ground cinnamon
- ✓ 1/2 tsp vanilla extract
- ✓ 1/2 cup dried figs, chopped

Directions:

- ❖ Place the quinoa, almond milk, sugar, salt, nutmeg, cinnamon and vanilla extract in a saucepan.
- ❖ Bring it to a boil over medium-high heat. Turn the heat to a simmer and let it cook for about 20 minutes; fluff with a fork.
- ❖ Divide between three serving bowls and garnish with dried figs. Enjoy

209) BREAD PUDDING WITH RAISINS

Preparation Time: 1 hour

Servings: 4

Ingredients:

- ✓ 4 cups day-old bread, cubed
- ✓ 1 cup brown sugar
- ✓ 4 cups coconut milk
- ✓ 1/2 tsp vanilla extract
- ✓ 1 tsp ground cinnamon
- ✓ 2 tbsp rum
- ✓ 1/2 cup raisins

Directions:

- ❖ Start by preheating your oven to 360 degrees F. Lightly oil a casserole dish with a nonstick cooking spray.
- ❖ Place the cubed bread in the prepared casserole dish.
- ❖ In a mixing bowl, thoroughly combine the sugar, milk, vanilla, cinnamon, rum and raisins. Pour the custard evenly over the bread cubes.
- ❖ Let it soak for about 15 minutes.
- ❖ Bake in the preheated oven for about 45 minutes or until the top is golden and set. Enjoy

210) BULGUR WHEAT SALAD

Preparation Time: 25 minutes   **Servings: 4**

Ingredients:

- ✓ 1 cup bulgur wheat
- ✓ 1 ½ cups vegetable broth
- ✓ 1 tsp sea salt
- ✓ 1 tsp fresh ginger, minced
- ✓ 4 tbsp olive oil
- ✓ 1 onion, chopped
- ✓ 8 ounces canned garbanzo beans, drained
- ✓ 2 large roasted peppers, sliced
- ✓ 2 tbsp fresh parsley, roughly chopped

Directions:

- ❖ In a deep saucepan, bring the bulgur wheat and vegetable broth to a simmer; let it cook, covered, for 12 to 13 minutes.
- ❖ Let it stand for about 10 minutes and fluff with a fork.
- ❖ Add the remaining ingredients to the cooked bulgur wheat; serve at room temperature or well-chilled. Enjoy

211) RYE PORRIDGE WITH BLUEBERRY TOPPING

Preparation Time: 15 minutes   **Servings: 3**

Ingredients:

- ✓ 1 cup rye flakes
- ✓ 1 cup water
- ✓ 1 cup coconut milk
- ✓ 1 cup fresh blueberries
- ✓ 1 tbsp coconut oil
- ✓ 6 dates, pitted

Directions:

- ❖ Add the rye flakes, water and coconut milk to a deep saucepan; bring to a boil over medium-high. Turn the heat to a simmer and let it cook for 5 to 6 minutes.
- ❖ In a blender or food processor, puree the blueberries with the coconut oil and dates.
- ❖ Ladle into three bowls and garnish with the blueberry topping.
- ❖ Enjoy

212) COCONUT SORGHUM PORRIDGE

Preparation Time: 15 minutes   **Servings: 2**

Ingredients:

- ✓ 1/2 cup sorghum
- ✓ 1 cup water
- ✓ 1/2 cup coconut milk
- ✓ 1/4 tsp grated nutmeg
- ✓ 1/4 tsp ground cloves
- ✓ 1/2 tsp ground cinnamon
- ✓ Kosher salt, to taste
- ✓ 2 tbsp agave syrup
- ✓ 2 tbsp coconut flakes

Directions:

- ❖ Place the sorghum, water, milk, nutmeg, cloves, cinnamon and kosher salt in a saucepan; simmer gently for about 15 minutes.
- ❖ Spoon the porridge into serving bowls. Top with agave syrup and coconut flakes. Enjoy

213)   MUM'S AROMATIC RICE

Preparation Time: 20 minutes

Servings: 4

Ingredients:

- ✓ 3 tbsp olive oil
- ✓ 1 tsp garlic, minced
- ✓ 1 tsp dried oregano
- ✓ 1 tsp dried rosemary
- ✓ 1 bay leaf
- ✓ 1 ½ cups white rice
- ✓ 2 ½ cups vegetable broth
- ✓ Sea salt and cayenne pepper, to taste

Directions:

- ❖ In a saucepan, heat the olive oil over a moderately high flame. Add in the garlic, oregano, rosemary and bay leaf; sauté for about 1 minute or until aromatic.
- ❖ Add in the rice and broth. Bring to a boil; immediately turn the heat to a gentle simmer.
- ❖ Cook for about 15 minutes or until all the liquid has absorbed. Fluff the rice with a fork, season with salt and pepper and serve immediately.
- ❖ Enjoy

214)   EVERYDAY SAVORY GRITS

Preparation Time: 35 minutes

Servings: 4

Ingredients:

- ✓ 2 tbsp vegan butter
- ✓ 1 sweet onion, chopped
- ✓ 1 tsp garlic, minced
- ✓ 4 cups water
- ✓ 1 cup stone-ground grits
- ✓ Sea salt and cayenne pepper, to taste

Directions:

- ❖ In a saucepan, melt the vegan butter over medium-high heat. Once hot, cook the onion for about 3 minutes or until tender.
- ❖ Add in the garlic and continue to sauté for 30 seconds more or until aromatic; reserve.
- ❖ Bring the water to a boil over a moderately high heat. Stir in the grits, salt and pepper. Turn the heat to a simmer, cover and continue to cook, for about 30 minutes or until cooked through.
- ❖ Stir in the sautéed mixture and serve warm. Enjoy

215)   GREEK-STYLE BARLEY SALAD

Preparation Time: 35 minutes

Servings: 4

Ingredients:

- ✓ 1 cup pearl barley
- ✓ 2 ¾ cups vegetable broth
- ✓ 2 tbsp apple cider vinegar
- ✓ 4 tbsp extra-virgin olive oil
- ✓ 2 bell peppers, seeded and diced
- ✓ 1 shallot, chopped
- ✓ 2 ounces sun-dried tomatoes in oil, chopped
- ✓ 1/2 green olives, pitted and sliced
- ✓ 2 tbsp fresh cilantro, roughly chopped

Directions:

- ❖ Bring the barley and broth to a boil over medium-high heat; now, turn the heat to a simmer.
- ❖ Continue to simmer for about 30 minutes until all the liquid has absorbed; fluff with a fork.
- ❖ Toss the barley with the vinegar, olive oil, peppers, shallots, sun-dried tomatoes and olives; toss to combine well.
- ❖ Garnish with fresh cilantro and serve at room temperature or well-chilled. Enjoy

216)   SWEET MAIZE MEAL PORRIDGE

Preparation Time: 15 minutes   Servings: 2

Ingredients:

- ✓ 2 cups water
- ✓ 1/2 cup maize meal
- ✓ 1/4 tsp ground allspice
- ✓ 1/4 tsp salt
- ✓ 2 tbsp brown sugar
- ✓ 2 tbsp almond butter

Directions:

- ❖ In a saucepan, bring the water to a boil; then, gradually add in the maize meal and turn the heat to a simmer.
- ❖ Add in the ground allspice and salt. Let it cook for 10 minutes.
- ❖ Add in the brown sugar and almond butter and gently stir to combine. Enjoy

217)   DAD'S MILLET MUFFINS

Preparation Time: 20 minutes   Servings: 8

Ingredients:

- ✓ 2 cup whole-wheat flour
- ✓ 1/2 cup millet
- ✓ 2 tsp baking powder
- ✓ 1/2 tsp salt
- ✓ 1 cup coconut milk
- ✓ 1/2 cup coconut oil, melted
- ✓ 1/2 cup agave nectar
- ✓ 1/2 tsp ground cinnamon
- ✓ 1/4 tsp ground cloves
- ✓ A pinch of grated nutmeg
- ✓ 1/2 cup dried apricots, chopped

Directions:

- ❖ Begin by preheating your oven to 400 degrees F. Lightly oil a muffin tin with a nonstick oil.
- ❖ In a mixing bowl, mix all dry ingredients. In a separate bowl, mix the wet ingredients. Stir the milk mixture into the flour mixture; mix just until evenly moist and do not overmix your batter.
- ❖ Fold in the apricots and scrape the batter into the prepared muffin cups.
- ❖ Bake the muffins in the preheated oven for about 15 minutes, or until a tester inserted in the center of your muffin comes out dry and clean.
- ❖ Let it stand for 10 minutes on a wire rack before unmolding and serving. Enjoy

218)   GINGER BROWN RICE

Preparation Time: 30 minutes   Servings: 4

Ingredients:

- ✓ 1 ½ cups brown rice, rinsed
- ✓ 2 tbsp olive oil
- ✓ 1 (1-inch) piece ginger, peeled and minced
- ✓ 1/2 tsp cumin seeds
- ✓ Sea salt and ground

Directions:

- ❖ Place the brown rice in a saucepan and cover with cold water by 2 inches. Bring to a boil.
- ❖ Turn the heat to a simmer and continue to cook for

✓ 1 tsp garlic, minced

black pepper, to taste

about 30 minutes or until tender.

❖ In a sauté pan, heat the olive oil over medium-high heat. Once hot, cook the garlic, ginger and cumin seeds until aromatic.

❖ Stir the garlic/ginger mixture into the hot rice; season with salt and pepper and serve immediately

219) CHILI BEAN AND BROWN RICE TORTILLAS

Preparation Time: 50 minutes

Servings: 4

Ingredients:

✓ 1 cups brown rice
✓ Salt and black pepper to taste
✓ 1 tbsp olive oil
✓ 1 medium red onion, chopped
✓ 1 green bell pepper, diced
✓ 2 garlic cloves, minced
✓ 1 tbsp chili powder
✓ 1 tsp cumin powder
✓ 1/8 tsp red chili flakes
✓ 1 (15 oz) can black beans, rinsed
✓ 4 whole-wheat flour tortillas, warmed
✓ 1 cup salsa
✓ 1 cup coconut cream for topping
✓ 1 cup grated plant-based cheddar

Directions:

❖ Add 2 cups of water and brown rice to a medium pot, season with some salt, and cook over medium heat until the water absorbs and the rice is tender, 15 to 20 minutes.

❖ Heat the olive oil in a medium skillet over medium heat and sauté the onion, bell pepper, and garlic until softened and fragrant, 3 minutes.

❖ Mix in the chili powder, cumin powder, red chili flakes, and season with salt and black pepper. Cook for 1 minute or until the food releases fragrance. Stir in the brown rice, black beans, and allow warming through, 3 minutes. Lay the tortillas on a clean, flat surface and divide the rice mixture in the center of each. Top with the salsa, coconut cream, and plant cheddar cheese. Fold the sides and ends of the tortillas over the filling to secure. Serve immediately

220)   CASHEW BUTTERED QUESADILLAS WITH LEAFY GREENS

Preparation Time: 30 minutes

Servings: 4

Ingredients:

- ✓ 3 tbsp flax seed powder
- ✓ ½ cup cashew cream cheese
- ✓ 1 ½ tsp psyllium husk powder
- ✓ 1 tbsp coconut flour
- ✓ ½ tsp salt
- ✓ 1 tbsp cashew butter
- ✓ 5 oz grated plant-based cheddar
- ✓ 1 oz leafy greens

Directions:

- ❖ Preheat oven to 400 F.
- ❖ In a bowl, mix flax seed powder with ½ cup water and allow sitting to thicken for 5 minutes. Whisk cashew cream cheese into the vegan "flax egg" until the batter is smooth. In another bowl, combine psyllium husk powder, coconut flour, and salt. Add the flour mixture to the flax egg batter and fold in until incorporated. Allow sitting for a few minutes. Line a baking sheet with wax paper and pour in the mixture. Spread and bake for 5-7 minutes. Slice into 8 pieces. Set aside.
- ❖ For the filling, spoon a little cashew butter into a skillet and place a tortilla in the pan. Sprinkle with some plant-based cheddar cheese, leafy greens, and cover with another tortilla. Brown each side of the quesadilla for 1 minute or until the cheese melts. Transfer to a plate. Repeat assembling the quesadillas using the remaining cashew butter. Serve

221)   ASPARAGUS WITH CREAMY PUREE

Preparation Time: 15 minutes

Servings: 4

Ingredients:

- ✓ 4 tbsp flax seed powder
- ✓ 2 oz plant butter, melted
- ✓ 3 oz cashew cream cheese
- ✓ ½ cup coconut cream
- ✓ Powdered chili pepper to taste
- ✓ 1 tbsp olive oil
- ✓ ½ lb asparagus, hard stalks removed
- ✓ 3 oz plant butter
- ✓ Juice of ½ a lemon

Directions:

- ❖ In a safe microwave bowl, mix the flax seed powder with ½ cup water and set aside to thicken for 5 minutes. Warm the vegan "flax egg" in the microwave for 1-2 minutes, then pour it into a blender. Add in plant butter, cashew cream cheese, coconut cream, salt, and chili pepper. Puree until smooth.
- ❖ Heat olive oil in a saucepan and roast the asparagus until lightly charred. Season with salt and black pepper and set aside. Melt plant butter in a frying pan until nutty and golden brown. Stir in lemon juice and pour the mixture into a sauce cup. Spoon the creamy blend into the center of four serving plates and use the back of the spoon to spread out lightly. Top with the asparagus and drizzle the lemon butter on top. Serve immediately

222) **KALE MUSHROOM GALETTE**

Preparation Time: 35 minutes

Servings: 4

Ingredients:

- ✓ 1 tbsp flax seed powder
- ✓ ½ cup grated plant-based mozzarella
- ✓ 1 tbsp plant butter
- ✓ ½ cup almond flour
- ✓ ¼ cup coconut flour
- ✓ ½ tsp onion powder
- ✓ 1 tsp baking powder
- ✓ 3 oz cashew cream cheese, softened
- ✓ 1 garlic clove, finely minced
- ✓ Salt and black pepper to taste
- ✓ 1 cup kale, chopped
- ✓ 2 oz cremini mushrooms, sliced
- ✓ 2 oz grated plant-based mozzarella
- ✓ 1 oz grated plant-based Parmesan
- ✓ Olive oil for brushing

Directions:

- ❖ Preheat oven to 375 F. Line a baking sheet with parchment paper and grease with cooking spray.
- ❖ In a bowl, mix flax seed powder with 3 tbsp water and allow sitting to thicken for 5 minutes. Place a pot over low heat, add in plant-based mozzarella and plant butter, and melt both whiles stirring continuously; remove. Stir in almond and coconut flours, onion powder, baking powder, and ¼ tsp salt. Pour in the vegan "flax egg" and combine until a quite sticky dough forms. Transfer dough to the baking sheet and cover with another parchment paper. Use a rolling pin to flatten into a 12-inch circle.
- ❖ After, remove the parchment paper and spread the cashew cream cheese on the dough, leaving about a 2-inch border around the edges. Sprinkle with garlic, salt, and black pepper. Spread kale on top of the cheese, followed by the mushrooms. Sprinkle the plant-based mozzarella and plant-based Parmesan cheese on top. Fold the ends of the crust over the filling and brush with olive oil. Bake until the cheese has melted and the crust golden brown, about 25-30 minutes. Slice and serve with arugula salad

223) FOCACCIA WITH MIXED MUSHROOMS

Preparation Time: 35 minutes

Servings: 4

Ingredients:

- ✓ 2 tbsp flax seed powder
- ✓ ½ cup tofu mayonnaise
- ✓ ¾ cup almond flour
- ✓ 1 tbsp psyllium husk powder
- ✓ 1 tsp baking powder
- ✓ 2 oz mixed mushrooms, sliced
- ✓ 1 tbsp plant-based basil pesto
- ✓ 2 tbsp olive oil
- ✓ Salt and black pepper to taste
- ✓ ½ cup coconut cream
- ✓ ¾ cup grated plant-based Parmesan

Directions:

- ❖ Preheat oven to 350 F.
- ❖ Combine flax seed powder with 6 tbsp water and allow sitting to thicken for 5 minutes. Whisk in tofu mayonnaise, almond flour, psyllium husk powder, baking powder, and salt. Allow sitting for 5 minutes. Pour the batter into a baking sheet and spread out with a spatula. Bake for 10 minutes.
- ❖ In a bowl, mix mushrooms with pesto, olive oil, salt, and black pepper. Remove the crust from the oven and spread the coconut cream on top. Add the mushroom mixture and plant-based Parmesan cheese. Bake the pizza further until the cheese has melted, 5-10 minutes. Slice and serve with salad

224) SEITAN CAKES WITH BROCCOLI MASH

Preparation Time: 30 minutes

Servings: 4

Ingredients:

- ✓ 1 tbsp flax seed powder
- ✓ 1 ½ lb crumbled seitan
- ✓ ½ white onion
- ✓ 2 oz olive oil
- ✓ 1 lb broccoli
- ✓ 5 oz cold plant butter
- ✓ 2 oz grated plant-based Parmesan
- ✓ 4 oz plant butter, room temperature
- ✓ 2 tbsp lemon juice

Directions:

- ❖ Preheat oven to 220 F. In a bowl, mix the flax seed powder with 3 tbsp water and allow sitting to thicken for 5 minutes. When the vegan "flax egg" is ready, add in crumbled seitan, white onion, salt, and pepper. Mix and mold out 6-8 cakes out of the mixture. Melt plant butter in a skillet and fry the patties on both sides until golden brown. Remove onto a wire rack to cool slightly.
- ❖ Pour salted water into a pot, bring to a boil, and add in broccoli. Cook until the broccoli is tender but not too soft. Drain and transfer to a bowl. Add in cold plant butter, plant-based Parmesan, salt, and pepper. Puree the ingredients until smooth and creamy. Set aside. Mix the soft plant butter with lemon juice, salt, and pepper in a bowl. Serve the seitan cakes with the broccoli mash and lemon butter

225)   SPICY CHEESE WITH TOFU BALLS

Preparation Time: 40 minutes   **Servings: 4**

Ingredients:

- ✓ 1/3 cup tofu mayonnaise
- ✓ ¼ cup pickled jalapenos
- ✓ 1 tsp paprika powder
- ✓ 1 tbsp mustard powder
- ✓ 1 pinch cayenne pepper
- ✓ 4 oz grated plant-based cheddar
- ✓ 1 tbsp flax seed powder
- ✓ 2 ½ cup crumbled tofu
- ✓ 2 tbsp plant butter

Directions:

- ❖ In a bowl, mix tofu mayonnaise, jalapeños, paprika, mustard powder, cayenne powder, and plant-based cheddar cheese; set aside. In another bowl, combine flax seed powder with 3 tbsp water and allow absorbing for 5 minutes. Add the vegan "flax egg" to the cheese mixture, crumbled tofu, salt, and pepper and combine well. Form meatballs out of the mix. Melt plant butter in a skillet and fry the tofu balls until browned. Serve the tofu balls with roasted cauliflower mash

226)   QUINOA ANDVEGGIE BURGERS

Preparation Time: 35 minutes   **Servings: 4**

Ingredients:

- ✓ 1 cup quick-cooking quinoa
- ✓ 1 tbsp olive oil
- ✓ 1 shallot, chopped
- ✓ 2 tbsp chopped fresh celery
- ✓ 1 garlic clove, minced
- ✓ 1 (15 oz) can pinto beans, drained
- ✓ 2 tbsp whole-wheat flour
- ✓ ¼ cup chopped fresh basil
- ✓ 2 tbsp pure maple syrup
- ✓ 4 whole-grain hamburger buns, split
- ✓ 4 small lettuce leaves for topping
- ✓ ½ cup tofu mayonnaise for topping

Directions:

- ❖ Cook the quinoa with 2 cups of water in a medium pot until the liquid absorbs, 10 to 15 minutes. Heat the olive oil in a medium skillet over medium heat and sauté the shallot, celery, and garlic until softened and fragrant, 3 minutes.
- ❖ Transfer the quinoa and shallot mixture to a medium bowl and add the pinto beans, flour, basil, maple syrup, salt, and black pepper. Mash and mold 4 patties out of the mixture and set aside.
- ❖ Heat a grill pan to medium heat and lightly grease with cooking spray. Cook the patties on both sides until light brown, compacted, and cooked through, 10 minutes. Place the patties between the burger buns and top with the lettuce and tofu mayonnaise. Serve

227) **BAKED TOFU WITH ROASTED PEPPERS**

Preparation Time: 20 minutes

Servings: 4

Ingredients:

- ✓ 3 oz cashew cream cheese
- ✓ ¾ cup tofu mayonnaise
- ✓ 2 oz cucumber, diced
- ✓ 1 large tomato, chopped
- ✓ 2 tsp dried parsley
- ✓ 4 medium orange bell peppers
- ✓ 2 ½ cups cubed tofu
- ✓ 1 tbsp melted plant butter
- ✓ 1 tsp dried basil

Directions:

- ❖ Preheat the oven's broiler to 450 F and line a baking sheet with parchment paper. In a salad bowl, combine cashew cream cheese, tofu mayonnaise, cucumber, tomato, salt, pepper, and parsley. Refrigerate.
- ❖ Arrange the bell peppers and tofu on the baking sheet, drizzle with melted plant butter, and season with basil, salt, and pepper. Bake for 10-15 minutes or until the peppers have charred lightly and the tofu browned. Remove from the oven and serve with the salad

228) **ZOODLE BOLOGNESE**

Preparation Time: 45 minutes

Servings: 4

Ingredients:

- ✓ 3 oz olive oil
- ✓ 1 white onion, chopped
- ✓ 1 garlic clove, minced
- ✓ 3 oz carrots, chopped
- ✓ 3 cups crumbled tofu
- ✓ 2 tbsp tomato paste
- ✓ 1 ½ cups crushed tomatoes
- ✓ Salt and black pepper to taste
- ✓ 1 tbsp dried basil
- ✓ 1 tbsp vegan Worcestershire sauce
- ✓ 2 lb zucchini, spiralized
- ✓ 2 tbsp plant butter

Directions:

- ❖ Pour olive oil into a saucepan and heat over medium heat. Add in onion, garlic, and carrots and sauté for 3 minutes or until the onions are soft and the carrots caramelized. Pour in tofu, tomato paste, tomatoes, salt, pepper, basil, and Worcestershire sauce. Stir and cook for 15 minutes. Mix in some water if the mixture is too thick and simmer further for 20 minutes. Melt plant butter in a skillet and toss in the zoodles quickly, about 1 minute. Season with salt and black pepper. Divide into serving plates and spoon the Bolognese on top. Serve immediately

229)   ZUCCHINI BOATS WITH VEGAN CHEESE

Preparation Time: 40 minutes

Servings: 2

Ingredients:

- ✓ 1 medium-sized zucchini
- ✓ 4 tbsp plant butter
- ✓ 2 garlic cloves, minced
- ✓ 1 ½ oz baby kale
- ✓ Salt and black pepper to taste
- ✓ 2 tbsp unsweetened tomato sauce
- ✓ 1 cup grated plant-based mozzarella
- ✓ Olive oil for drizzling

Directions:

- ❖ Preheat oven to 375 F.
- ❖ Use a knife to slice the zucchini in halves and scoop out the pulp with a spoon into a plate. Keep the flesh. Grease a baking sheet with cooking spray and place the zucchini boats on top. Put the plant butter in a skillet and melt over medium heat.
- ❖ Sauté the garlic for 1 minute. Add in kale and zucchini pulp. Cook until the kale wilts; season with salt and black pepper. Spoon tomato sauce into the boats and spread to coat the bottom evenly. Then, spoon the kale mixture into the zucchinis and sprinkle with the plant-based mozzarella cheese. Bake for 20-25 minutes. Serve immediately

230)   ROASTED BUTTERNUT SQUASH WITH CHIMICHURRI

Preparation Time: 15 minutes

Servings: 4

Ingredients:

- ✓ Zest and juice of 1 lemon
- ✓ ½ medium red bell pepper, chopped
- ✓ 1 jalapeno pepper, chopped
- ✓ 1 cup olive oil
- ✓ ½ cup chopped fresh parsley
- ✓ 2 garlic cloves, minced
- ✓ 1 lb butternut squash
- ✓ 1 tbsp plant butter, melted
- ✓ 3 tbsp toasted pine nuts

Directions:

- ❖ In a bowl, add the lemon zest and juice, red bell pepper, jalapeno, olive oil, parsley, garlic, salt, and black pepper. Use an immersion blender to grind the ingredients until your desired consistency is achieved; set aside the chimichurri.
- ❖ Slice the butternut squash into rounds and remove the seeds. Drizzle with the plant butter and season with salt and black pepper. Preheat a grill pan over medium heat and cook the squash for 2 minutes on each side or until browned. Remove the squash to serving plates, scatter the pine nuts on top, and serve with the chimichurri and red cabbage salad

231) SWEET AND SPICY BRUSSEL SPROUT STIR-FRY

Preparation Time: 15 minutes   **Servings: 4**

Ingredients:

- ✓ 4 oz plant butter + more to taste
- ✓ 4 shallots, chopped
- ✓ 1 tbsp apple cider vinegar
- ✓ Salt and black pepper to taste
- ✓ 1 lb Brussels sprouts
- ✓ Hot chili sauce

Directions:

- ❖ Put the plant butter in a saucepan and melt over medium heat. Pour in the shallots and sauté for 2 minutes, to caramelize and slightly soften. Add the apple cider vinegar, salt, and black pepper. Stir and reduce the heat to cook the shallots further with continuous stirring, about 5 minutes. Transfer to a plate after.
- ❖ Trim the Brussel sprouts and cut in halves. Leave the small ones as wholes. Pour the Brussel sprouts into the saucepan and stir-fry with more plant butter until softened but al dente. Season with salt and black pepper, stir in the onions and hot chili sauce, and heat for a few seconds. Serve immediately

232) BLACK BEAN BURGERS WITH BBQ SAUCE

Preparation Time: 20 minutes   **Servings: 4**

Ingredients:

- ✓ 3 (15 oz) cans black beans, drained
- ✓ 2 tbsp whole-wheat flour
- ✓ 2 tbsp quick-cooking oats
- ✓ ¼ cup chopped fresh basil
- ✓ 2 tbsp pure barbecue sauce
- ✓ 1 garlic clove, minced
- ✓ Salt and black pepper to taste
- ✓ 4 whole-grain hamburger buns, split
- ✓ For topping:
- ✓ Red onion slices
- ✓ Tomato slices
- ✓ Fresh basil leaves
- ✓ Additional barbecue sauce

Directions:

- ❖ In a medium bowl, mash the black beans and mix in the flour, oats, basil, barbecue sauce, garlic salt, and black pepper until well combined. Mold 4 patties out of the mixture and set aside.
- ❖ Heat a grill pan to medium heat and lightly grease with cooking spray. Cook the bean patties on both sides until light brown and cooked through, 10 minutes. Place the patties between the burger buns and top with the onions, tomatoes, basil, and some barbecue sauce. Serve warm

233)   CREAMY BRUSSELS SPROUTS BAKE

Preparation Time: 26 minutes   **Servings: 4**

Ingredients:

- ✓ 3 tbsp plant butter
- ✓ 1 cup tempeh, cut into 1-inch cubes
- ✓ 1 ½ lb halved Brussels sprouts
- ✓ 5 garlic cloves, minced
- ✓ 1 ¼ cups coconut cream
- ✓ 10 oz grated plant-based mozzarella
- ✓ ¼ cup grated plant-based Parmesan
- ✓ Salt and black pepper to taste

Directions:

- ❖ Preheat oven to 400 F.
- ❖ Melt the plant butter in a large skillet over medium heat and fry the tempeh cubes until browned on both sides, about 6 minutes. Remove onto a plate and set aside. Pour the Brussels sprouts and garlic into the skillet and sauté until fragrant.
- ❖ Mix in coconut cream and simmer for 4 minutes. Add tempeh cubes and combine well. Pour the sauté into a baking dish, sprinkle with plant-based mozzarella cheese, and plant-based Parmesan cheese. Bake for 10 minutes or until golden brown on top. Serve with tomato salad

234)   BASIL PESTO SEITAN PANINI

Preparation Time: 15 minutes+ cooling time   **Servings: 4**

Ingredients:

- ✓ For the seitan:
- ✓ 2/3 cup basil pesto
- ✓ ½ lemon, juiced
- ✓ 1 garlic clove, minced
- ✓ 1/8 tsp salt
- ✓ 1 cup chopped seitan
- ✓ For the panini:
- ✓ 3 tbsp basil pesto
- ✓ 8 thick slices whole-wheat ciabatta
- ✓ Olive oil for brushing
- ✓ 8 slices plant-based mozzarella
- ✓ 1 yellow bell pepper, chopped
- ✓ ¼ cup grated plant Parmesan cheese

Directions:

- ❖ In a medium bowl, mix the pesto, lemon juice, garlic, and salt. Add the seitan and coat well with the marinade. Cover with plastic wrap and marinate in the refrigerator for 30 minutes.
- ❖ Preheat a large skillet over medium heat and remove the seitan from the fridge. Cook the seitan in the skillet until brown and cooked through, 2-3 minutes. Turn the heat off.
- ❖ Preheat a panini press to medium heat. In a small bowl, mix the pesto in the inner parts of two slices of bread. On the outer parts, apply some olive oil and place a slice with (the olive oil side down) in the press. Lay 2 slices of plant-based mozzarella cheese on the bread, spoon some seitan on top. Sprinkle with some bell pepper and some plant-based Parmesan cheese. Cover with another bread slice.
- ❖ Close the press and grill the bread for 1 to 2 minutes. Flip the bread, and grill further for 1 minute or until the cheese melts and golden brown on both sides. Serve warm

235)   SWEET OATMEAL "GRITS"

Preparation Time: 20 minutes

Servings: 4

Ingredients:

- ✓ 1 ½ cups steel-cut oats, soaked overnight
- ✓ 1 cup almond milk
- ✓ 2 cups water
- ✓ A pinch of grated nutmeg
- ✓ A pinch of ground cloves
- ✓ A pinch of sea salt
- ✓ 4 tbsp almonds, slivered
- ✓ 6 dates, pitted and chopped
- ✓ 6 prunes, chopped

Directions:

- ❖ In a deep saucepan, bring the steel cut oats, almond milk and water to a boil.
- ❖ Add in the nutmeg, cloves and salt. Immediately turn the heat to a simmer, cover and continue to cook for about 15 minutes or until they've softened.
- ❖ Then, spoon the grits into four serving bowls; top them with the almonds, dates and prunes.
- ❖ Enjoy!

236)   FREEKEH BOWL WITH DRIED FIGS

Preparation Time: 35 minutes

Servings: 2

Ingredients:

- ✓ 1/2 cup freekeh, soaked for 30 minutes, drained
- ✓ 1 1/3 cups almond milk
- ✓ 1/4 tsp sea salt
- ✓ 1/4 tsp ground cloves
- ✓ 1/4 tsp ground cinnamon
- ✓ 4 tbsp agave syrup
- ✓ 2 ounces dried figs, chopped

Directions:

- ❖ Place the freekeh, milk, sea salt, ground cloves and cinnamon in a saucepan. Bring to a boil over medium-high heat.
- ❖ Immediately turn the heat to a simmer for 30 to 35 minutes, stirring occasionally to promote even cooking.
- ❖ Stir in the agave syrup and figs. Ladle the porridge into individual bowls and serve. Enjoy

237)   CORNMEAL PORRIDGE WITH MAPLE SYRUP

Preparation Time: 20 minutes

Servings: 4

Ingredients:

- ✓ 2 cups water
- ✓ 2 cups almond milk
- ✓ 1 cinnamon stick
- ✓ 1 vanilla bean
- ✓ 1 cup yellow cornmeal
- ✓ 1/2 cup maple syrup

Directions:

- ❖ In a saucepan, bring the water and almond milk to a boil. Add in the cinnamon stick and vanilla bean.
- ❖ Gradually add in the cornmeal, stirring continuously; turn the heat to a simmer. Let it simmer for about 15 minutes.
- ❖ Drizzle the maple syrup over the porridge and serve warm. Enjoy

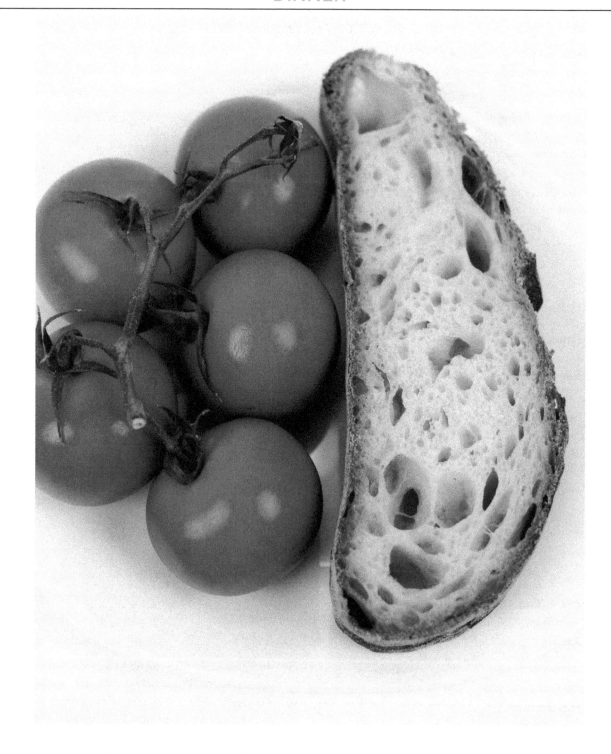

238) MATCHA-INFUSED TOFU RICE

Preparation Time: 35 minutes

Servings: 4

Ingredients:

- ✓ 4 matcha tea bags
- ✓ 1 ½ cups brown rice
- ✓ 2 tbsp canola oil
- ✓ 8 oz extra-firm tofu, chopped
- ✓ 3 green onions, minced
- ✓ 2 cups snow peas, cut diagonally
- ✓ 1 tbsp fresh lemon juice
- ✓ 1 tsp grated lemon zest
- ✓ Salt and black pepper to taste

Directions:

- ❖ Boil 3 cups water in a pot. Place in the tea bags and turn the heat off. Let sit for 7 minutes. Discard the bags. Wash the rice and put it into the tea. Cook for 20 minutes over medium heat. Drain and set aside.
- ❖ Heat the oil in a skillet over medium heat. Fry the tofu for 5 minutes until golden. Stir in green onions and snow peas and cook for another 3 minutes. Mix in lemon juice and lemon zest. Place the rice in a serving bowl and mix in the tofu mixture. Adjust the seasoning with salt and pepper. Serve right away

239) CHINESE FRIED RICE

Preparation Time: 20 minutes

Servings: 4

Ingredients:

- ✓ 2 tbsp canola oil
- ✓ 1 onion, chopped
- ✓ 1 large carrot, chopped
- ✓ 1 head broccoli, cut into florets
- ✓ 2 garlic cloves, minced
- ✓ 2 tsp grated fresh ginger
- ✓ 3 green onions, minced
- ✓ 3 ½ cups cooked brown rice
- ✓ 1 cup frozen peas, thawed
- ✓ 3 tbsp soy sauce
- ✓ 2 tsp dry white wine
- ✓ 1 tbsp toasted sesame oil

Directions:

- ❖ Heat the oil in a skillet over medium heat. Place in onion, carrot, and broccoli, sauté for 5 minutes until tender. Add in garlic, ginger, and green onions and sauté for another 3 minutes. Stir in rice, peas, soy sauce, and white wine and cook for 5 minutes. Add in sesame oil, toss to combine. Serve right away

240) SAVORY SEITAN XAND BELL PEPPER RICE

Preparation Time: 35 minutes **Servings: 4**

Ingredients:

- ✓ 2 cups water
- ✓ 1 cup long-grain brown rice
- ✓ 2 tbsp olive oil
- ✓ 1 onion, chopped
- ✓ 2 garlic cloves, minced
- ✓ 8 oz seitan, chopped
- ✓ 1 green bell pepper, chopped
- ✓ 1 tsp dried basil
- ✓ ½ tsp ground fennel seeds
- ✓ ¼ tsp crushed red pepper
- ✓ Salt and black pepper to taste

Directions:

- ❖ Bring water to a boil in a pot. Place in rice and lower the heat. Simmer for 20 minutes.
- ❖ Heat the oil in a skillet over medium heat. Sauté the onion for 3 minutes until translucent. Add in the seitan and bell pepper and cook for another 5 minutes. Stir in basil, fennel, red pepper, salt, and black pepper. Once the rice is ready, remove it to a bowl. Add in seitan mixture and toss to combine. Serve

241) ASPARAGUS AND MUSHROOMS WITH MASHED POTATOES

Preparation Time: 60 minutes **Servings: 4**

Ingredients:

- ✓ 5 large portobello mushrooms, stems removed
- ✓ 6 potatoes, chopped
- ✓ 4 garlic cloves, minced
- ✓ 2 tsp olive oil
- ✓ ½ cup non-dairy milk
- ✓ 2 tbsp nutritional yeast
- ✓ Sea salt to taste
- ✓ 7 cups asparagus, chopped
- ✓ 3 tsp coconut oil
- ✓ 2 tbsp nutritional yeast

Directions:

- ❖ Place the chopped potatoes in a pot and cover with salted water. Cook for 20 minutes.
- ❖ Heat oil in a skillet and sauté garlic for 1 minute. Once the potatoes are ready, drain them and reserve the water. Transfer to a bowl and mash them with some hot water, garlic, milk, yeast, and salt.
- ❖ Preheat your grill to medium. Grease the mushrooms with cooking spray and season with salt. Arrange the mushrooms face down and grill for 10 minutes. After, grill the asparagus for about 10 minutes, turning often. Arrange the veggies in a serving platter. Add in the potato mash and serve

242) GREEN PEA AND LEMON COUSCOUS

Preparation Time: 15 minutes **Servings: 6**

Ingredients:

- ✓ 1 cup green peas
- ✓ 2 ¾ cups vegetable stock
- ✓ Juice and zest of 1 lemon
- ✓ 2 tbsp chopped fresh thyme
- ✓ 1 ½ cups couscous
- ✓ ¼ cup chopped fresh parsley

Directions:

- ❖ Pour the vegetable stock, lemon juice, thyme, salt, and pepper in a pot. Bring to a boil, then add in green peas and couscous. Turn the heat off and let sit covered for 5 minutes, until the liquid has absorbed. Fluff the couscous using a fork and mix in the lemon and parsley. Serve immediately

243) **CHIMICHURRI FUSILI WITH NAVY BEANS**

Preparation Time: 25 minutes

Servings: 4

Ingredients:

- ✓ 8 oz whole-wheat fusilli
- ✓ 1 ½ cups canned navy beans
- ✓ ½ cup chimichurri salsa
- ✓ 1 cup chopped tomatoes
- ✓ 1 red onion, chopped
- ✓ ½ cup chopped pitted black olives

Directions:

- ❖ n a large pot over medium heat, pour 8 cups of salted water. Bring to a boil and add in the pasta. Cook for 8-10 minutes, drain and let cool. Combine the pasta, beans, and chimichurri in a bowl. Toss to coat. Stir in tomato, red onion, and olives

244) **QUINOA AND CHICKPEA POT**

Preparation Time: 15 minutes

Servings: 2

Ingredients:

- ✓ 2 tsp olive oil
- ✓ 1 cup cooked quinoa
- ✓ 1 (15-oz) can chickpeas
- ✓ 1 bunch arugula chopped
- ✓ 1 tbsp soy
- ✓ Sea salt and black pepper to taste

Directions:

- ❖ Heat the oil in a skillet over medium heat. Stir in quinoa, chickpeas, and arugula and cook for 3-5 minutes until the arugula wilts. Pour in soy sauce, salt, and pepper. Toss to coat. Serve immediately

245) BUCKWHEAT PILAF WITH PINE NUTS

Preparation Time: 25 minutes   **Servings: 4**

Ingredients:

- ✓ 1 cup buckwheat groats
- ✓ 2 cups vegetable stock
- ✓ ¼ cup pine nuts
- ✓ 2 tbsp olive oil
- ✓ ½ onion, chopped
- ✓ ⅓ cup chopped fresh parsley

Directions:

- ❖ Put the groats and vegetable stock in a pot. Bring to a boil, then lower the heat and simmer for 15 minutes. Heat a skillet over medium heat. Place in the pine nuts and toast for 2-3 minutes, shaking often. Heat the oil in the same skillet and sauté the onion for 3 minutes until translucent.
- ❖ Once the groats are ready, fluff them using a fork. Mix in pine nuts, onion, and parsley. Sprinkle with salt and pepper. Serve

246)

247) ITALIAN HOLIDAY STUFFING

Preparation Time: 25 minutes   **Servings: 4**

Ingredients:

- ✓ ¼ cup plant butter
- ✓ 1 onion, chopped
- ✓ 2 celery stalks, sliced
- ✓ 1 cup button mushrooms, sliced
- ✓ 3 garlic cloves, minced
- ✓ ½ cup vegetable broth
- ✓ ½ cup raisins
- ✓ ½ cup chopped walnuts
- ✓ 2 cups cooked quinoa
- ✓ 1 tsp Italian seasoning
- ✓ Sea salt to taste
- ✓ Chopped fresh parsley

Directions:

- ❖ In a skillet over medium heat, melt the butter. Sauté the onion, garlic, celery, and mushrooms for 5 minutes until tender, stirring occasionally. Pour in broth, raisins, and walnuts. Bring to a boil, then lower the heat and simmer for 5 minutes. Stir in quinoa, Italian seasoning, and salt. Cook for another 4 minutes. Serve garnished with parsley

248) PRESSURE COOKER GREEN LENTILS

Preparation Time: 30 minutes   **Servings: 6**

Ingredients:

- ✓ 3 tbsp coconut oil
- ✓ 2 tbsp curry powder
- ✓ 1 tsp ground ginger
- ✓ 1 onion, chopped
- ✓ 2 garlic cloves, sliced
- ✓ 1 cup dried green lentils
- ✓ 3 cups water
- ✓ Salt and black pepper to taste

Directions:

- ❖ Set your IP to Sauté. Add in coconut oil, curry powder, ginger, onion, and garlic. Cook for 3 minutes. Stir in green lentils. Pour in water. Lock the lid and set the time to 10 minutes on High. Once ready, perform a natural pressure release for 10 minutes. Unlock the lid and season with salt and pepper. Serve

249)   CHERRY AND PISTACHIO BULGUR

Preparation Time: 45 minutes   **Servings: 4**

Ingredients:

- ✓ 1 tbsp plant butter
- ✓ 1 white onion, chopped
- ✓ 1 carrot, chopped
- ✓ 1 celery stalk, chopped
- ✓ 1 cup chopped mushrooms
- ✓ 1 ½ cups bulgur
- ✓ 4 cups vegetable broth
- ✓ 1 cup chopped dried cherries, soaked
- ✓ ½ cup chopped pistachios

Directions:

- ❖ Preheat oven to 375 F.
- ❖ Melt butter in a skillet over medium heat. Sauté the onion, carrot, and celery for 5 minutes until tender. Add in mushrooms and cook for 3 more minutes. Pour in bulgur and broth. Transfer to a casserole and bake covered for 30 minutes. Once ready, uncover and stir in cherries. Top with pistachios to serve

250)   MUSHROOM FRIED RICE

Preparation Time: 25 minutes   **Servings: 6**

Ingredients:

- ✓ 2 tbsp sesame oil
- ✓ 1 onion, chopped
- ✓ 1 carrot, chopped
- ✓ 1 cup okra, chopped
- ✓ 1 cup sliced shiitake mushrooms
- ✓ 2 garlic cloves, minced
- ✓ ¼ cup soy sauce
- ✓ 1 cups cooked brown rice
- ✓ 2 green onions, chopped

Directions:

- ❖ Heat the oil in a skillet over medium heat. Place in onion and carrot and cook for 3 minutes. Add in okra and mushrooms, cook for 5-7 minutes. Stir in garlic and cook for 30 seconds. Put in soy sauce and rice. Cook until hot. Add in green onions and stir. Serve warm

251)   BEAN AND BROWN RICE WITH ARTICHOKES

Preparation Time: 35 minutes   **Servings: 4**

Ingredients:

- ✓ 2 tbsp olive oil
- ✓ 3 garlic cloves, minced
- ✓ 1 cup artichokes hearts, chopped
- ✓ 1 tsp dried basil
- ✓ 1 ½ cups cooked navy beans
- ✓ 1 ½ cups long-grain brown rice
- ✓ 3 cups vegetable broth
- ✓ Salt and black pepper to taste
- ✓ 2 ripe grape tomatoes, quartered
- ✓ 2 tbsp minced fresh parsley

Directions:

- ❖ Heat the oil in a pot over medium heat. Sauté the garlic for 1 minute. Stir in artichokes, basil, navy beans, rice, and broth. Sprinkle with salt and pepper. Lower the heat and simmer for 20-25 minutes. Remove to a bowl and mix in tomatoes and parsley. Using a fork, fluff the rice and serve right away

252) **PRESSURE COOKER CELERY AND SPINACH CHICKPEAS**

Preparation Time: 50 minutes

Servings: 5

Ingredients:

- ✓ 1 cup chickpeas, soaked overnight
- ✓ 1 onion, chopped
- ✓ 2 garlic cloves, minced
- ✓ 1 celery stalk, chopped
- ✓ 2 tbsp olive oil
- ✓ 3 tsp ground cinnamon
- ✓ ½ tsp ground nutmeg
- ✓ 1 tbsp coconut oil
- ✓ 1 cup spinach, chopped

Directions:

- ❖ Place chickpeas in your IP with the onion, garlic, celery, olive oil, 2 cups water, cinnamon, and nutmeg.
- ❖ Lock the lid in place; set the time to 30 minutes on High. Once ready, perform a natural pressure release for 10 minutes. Unlock the lid and drain the excess water. Put back the chickpeas and stir in coconut oil and spinach. Set the pot to Sauté and cook for another 5 minutes

253) **VEGGIE PAELLA WITH LENTILS**

Preparation Time: 50 minutes

Servings: 4

Ingredients:

- ✓ 2 tbsp olive oil
- ✓ 1 onion, chopped
- ✓ 1 green bell pepper, chopped
- ✓ 2 garlic cloves, minced
- ✓ 1 (14.5-oz) can diced tomatoes
- ✓ 1 tbsp capers
- ✓ ¼ tsp crushed red pepper
- ✓ 1 ½ cups long-grain brown rice
- ✓ 3 cups vegetable broth
- ✓ 1 ½ cups cooked lentils, drained
- ✓ ¼ cup sliced pitted black olives
- ✓ 2 tbsp minced fresh parsley

Directions:

- ❖ Heat oil in a pot over medium heat and sauté onion, bell pepper, and garlic for 5 minutes. Stir in tomatoes, capers, red pepper, and salt. Cook for 5 minutes. Pour in the rice and broth. Bring to a boil, then lower the heat. Simmer for 20 minutes. Turn the heat off and mix in lentils. Serve garnished with olives and parsley

254)   **CURRY BEAN WITH ARTICHOKES**

Preparation Time: 25 minutes   **Servings: 4**

Ingredients:

- ✓ 1 (14.5-oz) can artichoke hearts, drained and quartered
- ✓ 1 tsp olive oil
- ✓ 1 small onion, diced
- ✓ 2 garlic cloves, minced
- ✓ 1 (14.5-oz) can cannellini beans
- ✓ 2 tsp curry powder
- ✓ ½ tsp ground coriander
- ✓ 1 (5.4-oz) can coconut milk
- ✓ Salt and black pepper to taste

Directions:

- ❖ Heat the oil in a skillet over medium heat. Sauté the onion and garlic for 3 minutes until translucent. Stir in beans, artichoke, curry powder, and coriander. Add in coconut milk. Bring to a boil, then lower the heat and simmer for 10 minutes. Serve

255)   **ENDIVE SLAW WITH OLIVES**

Preparation Time: 10 minutes   **Servings: 6**

Ingredients:

- ✓ 1 lb curly endive, chopped
- ✓ ⅓ cup vegan mayonnaise
- ✓ ¼ cup rice vinegar
- ✓ 2 tbsp vegan yogurt
- ✓ 1 tbsp pure date sugar
- ✓ 10 black olives for garnish
- ✓ ¼ tsp freshly ground black pepper
- ✓ ¼ tsp smoked paprika
- ✓ ¼ tsp chipotle powder

Directions:

- ❖ In a bowl, mix the mayonnaise, vinegar, yogurt, sugar, salt, pepper, paprika, and chipotle powder. Gently add in the curly endive and mix with a wooden spatula to coat. Top with black olives and serve

256)   **PAPRIKA CAULIFLOWER TACOS**

Preparation Time: 40 minutes   **Servings: 6**

Ingredients:

- ✓ 1 head cauliflower, cut into pieces
- ✓ 2 tbsp olive oil
- ✓ 2 tbsp whole-wheat flour
- ✓ 2 tbsp nutritional yeast
- ✓ 2 tsp paprika
- ✓ 1 tsp cayenne pepper
- ✓ Salt to taste
- ✓ 1 cups shredded watercress
- ✓ 2 cups cherry tomatoes, halved
- ✓ 2 carrots, grated
- ✓ ½ cup mango salsa
- ✓ ½ cup guacamole
- ✓ 8 small corn tortillas, warm
- ✓ 1 lime, cut into wedges

Directions:

- ❖ Preheat oven to 350 F.
- ❖ Brush the cauliflower with oil in a bowl. In another bowl, mix the flour, yeast, paprika, cayenne pepper, and salt. Pour into the cauliflower bowl and toss to coat. Spread the cauliflower on a greased baking sheet. Bake for 20-30 minutes.
- ❖ In a bowl, combine the watercress, cherry tomatoes, carrots, mango salsa, and guacamole. Once the cauliflower is ready, divide it between the tortillas, add the mango mixture, roll up and serve with lime wedges on the side

SNACKS

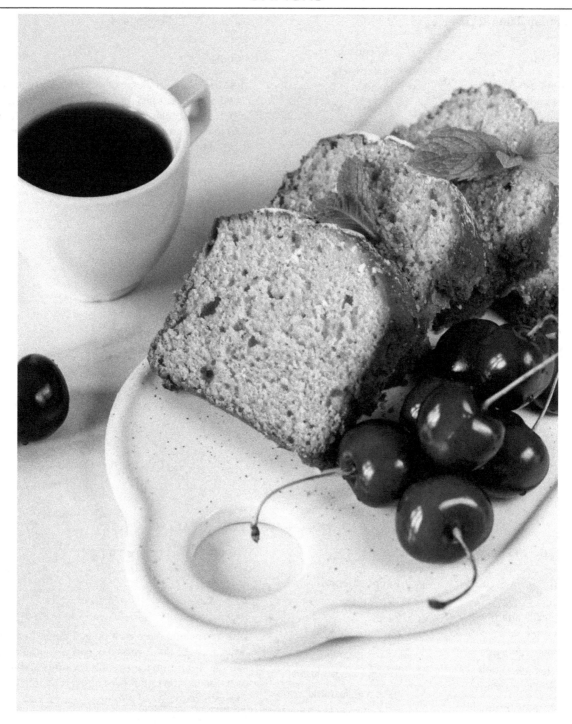

257)   FREEKEH SALAD WITH ZA'ATAR

Preparation Time: 35 minutes

Servings: 4

Ingredients:

- ✓ 1 cup freekeh
- ✓ 2 ½ cups water
- ✓ 1 cup grape tomatoes, halved
- ✓ 2 bell peppers, seeded and sliced
- ✓ 1 habanero pepper, seeded and sliced
- ✓ 1 onion, thinly sliced
- ✓ 2 tbsp fresh cilantro, chopped
- ✓ 2 tbsp fresh parsley, chopped
- ✓ 2 ounces green olives, pitted and sliced
- ✓ 1/4 cup extra-virgin olive oil
- ✓ 2 tbsp lemon juice
- ✓ 1 tsp deli mustard
- ✓ 1 tsp za'atar
- ✓ Sea salt and ground black pepper, to taste

Directions:

- ❖ Place the freekeh and water in a saucepan. Bring to a boil over medium-high heat.
- ❖ Immediately turn the heat to a simmer for 30 to 35 minutes, stirring occasionally to promote even cooking. Let it cool completely.
- ❖ Toss the cooked freekeh with the remaining ingredients. Toss to combine well.
- ❖ Enjoy

258)   VEGETABLE AMARANTH SOUP

Preparation Time: 30 minutes

Servings: 4

Ingredients:

- ✓ 2 tbsp olive oil
- ✓ 1 small shallot, chopped
- ✓ 1 carrot, trimmed and chopped
- ✓ 1 parsnip, trimmed and chopped
- ✓ 1 cup yellow squash, peeled and chopped
- ✓ 1 tsp fennel seeds
- ✓ 1 tsp celery seeds
- ✓ 1 tsp turmeric powder
- ✓ 1 bay laurel
- ✓ 1/2 cup amaranth
- ✓ 2 cups cream of celery soup
- ✓ 2 cups water
- ✓ 2 cups collard greens, torn into pieces
- ✓ Sea salt and ground black pepper, to taste

Directions:

- ❖ In a heavy-bottomed pot, heat the olive oil until sizzling. Once hot, sauté the shallot, carrot, parsnip and squash for 5 minutes or until just tender.
- ❖ Then, sauté the fennel seeds, celery seeds, turmeric powder and bay laurel for about 30 seconds, until aromatic.
- ❖ Add in the amaranth, soup and water. Turn the heat to a simmer. Cover and let it simmer for 15 to 18 minutes.
- ❖ Afterwards, add in the collard greens, season with salt and black pepper and continue to simmer for 5 minutes longer. Enjoy

259) POLENTA WITH MUSHROOMS AND CHICKPEAS

Preparation Time: 25 minutes

Servings: 4

Ingredients:

- ✓ 3 cups vegetable broth
- ✓ 1 cup yellow cornmeal
- ✓ 2 tbsp olive oil
- ✓ 1 onion, chopped
- ✓ 1 bell pepper, seeded and sliced
- ✓ 1 pound Cremini mushrooms, sliced
- ✓ 2 garlic cloves, minced
- ✓ 1/2 cup dry white wine
- ✓ 1/2 cup vegetable broth
- ✓ Kosher salt and freshly ground black pepper, to taste
- ✓ 1 tsp paprika
- ✓ 1 cup canned chickpeas, drained

Directions:

- ❖ In a medium saucepan, bring the vegetable broth to a boil over medium-high heat. Now, add in the cornmeal, whisking continuously to prevent lumps.
- ❖ Reduce the heat to a simmer. Continue to simmer, whisking periodically, for about 18 minutes, until the mixture has thickened.
- ❖ Meanwhile, heat the olive oil in a saucepan over a moderately high heat. Cook the onion and pepper for about 3 minutes or until just tender and fragrant.
- ❖ Add in the mushrooms and garlic; continue to sauté, gradually adding the wine and broth, for 4 more minutes or until cooked through. Season with salt, black pepper and paprika. Stir in the chickpeas.
- ❖ Spoon the mushroom mixture over your polenta and serve warm. Enjoy

260) TEFF SALAD WITH AVOCADO AND BEANS

Preparation Time: 20 minutes + chilling time

Servings: 2

Ingredients:

- ✓ 2 cups water
- ✓ 1/2 cup teff grain
- ✓ 1 tsp fresh lemon juice
- ✓ 3 tbsp vegan mayonnaise
- ✓ 1 tsp deli mustard
- ✓ 1 small avocado, pitted, peeled and sliced
- ✓ 1 small red onion, thinly sliced
- ✓ 1 small Persian cucumber, sliced
- ✓ 1/2 cup canned kidney beans, drained
- ✓ 2 cups baby spinach

Directions:

- ❖ In a deep saucepan, bring the water to a boil over high heat. Add in the teff grain and turn the heat to a simmer.
- ❖ Continue to cook, covered, for about 20 minutes or until tender. Let it cool completely.
- ❖ Add in the remaining ingredients and toss to combine. Serve at room temperature. Enjoy

261) OVERNIGHT OATMEAL WITH WALNUTS

Preparation Time: 5 minutes + chilling time

Servings: 3

Ingredients:

- ✓ 1 cup old-fashioned oats
- ✓ 3 tbsp chia seeds
- ✓ 1 ½ cups coconut milk
- ✓ 3 tsp agave syrup
- ✓ 1 tsp vanilla extract
- ✓ 1/2 tsp ground cinnamon
- ✓ 3 tbsp walnuts, chopped
- ✓ A pinch of salt
- ✓ A pinch of grated nutmeg

Directions:

- ❖ Divide the ingredients between three mason jars.
- ❖ Cover and shake to combine well. Let them sit overnight in your refrigerator.
- ❖ You can add some extra milk before serving. Enjoy

262) COLORFUL SPELT SALAD

Preparation Time: 50 minutes + chilling time

Servings: 4

Ingredients:

- ✓ 3 ½ cups water
- ✓ 1 cup dry spelt
- ✓ 1 cup canned kidney beans, drained
- ✓ 1 bell pepper, seeded and diced
- ✓ 2 medium tomatoes, diced
- ✓ 2 tbsp basil, chopped
- ✓ 2 tbsp parsley, chopped
- ✓ 2 tbsp mint, chopped
- ✓ 1/4 cup extra-virgin olive oil
- ✓ 1 tsp deli mustard
- ✓ 1 tbsp fresh lime juice
- ✓ 1 tbsp white vinegar
- ✓ Sea salt and cayenne pepper, to taste

Directions:

- ❖ Bring the water to a boil over medium-high heat. Now, add in the spelt, turn the heat to a simmer and continue to cook for approximately 50 minutes, until the spelt is tender. Drain and allow it to cool completely.
- ❖ Toss the spelt with the remaining ingredients; toss to combine well and place the salad in your refrigerator until ready to serve.
- ❖ Enjoy

263) POWERFUL TEFF BOWL WITH TAHINI SAUCE

Preparation Time: 20 minutes +

chilling time

Servings: 4

Ingredients:

- ✓ 3 cups water
- ✓ 1 cup teff
- ✓ 2 garlic cloves, pressed
- ✓ 4 tbsp tahini
- ✓ 2 tbsp tamari sauce
- ✓ 2 tbsp white vinegar
- ✓ 1 tsp agave nectar
- ✓ 1 tsp deli mustard
- ✓ 1 tsp Italian herb mix
- ✓ 1 cup canned chickpeas, drained
- ✓ 2 cups mixed greens
- ✓ 1 cup grape tomatoes, halved
- ✓ 1 Italian peppers, seeded and diced

Directions:

- ❖ In a deep saucepan, bring the water to a boil over high heat. Add in the teff grain and turn the heat to a simmer.
- ❖ Continue to cook, covered, for about 20 minutes or until tender. Let it cool completely and transfer to a salad bowl.
- ❖ In the meantime, mix the garlic, tahini, tamari sauce, vinegar, agave nectar, mustard and Italian herb mix; whisk until everything is well incorporated.
- ❖ Add the canned chickpeas, mixed greens, tomatoes and peppers to the salad bowl; toss to combine. Dress the salad and toss again. Serve at room temperature. Enjoy

264) POLENTA TOASTS WITH BALSAMIC ONIONS

Preparation Time: 25 minutes +

chilling time

Servings: 5

Ingredients:

- ✓ 3 cups vegetable broth
- ✓ 1 cup yellow cornmeal
- ✓ 4 tbsp vegan butter, divided
- ✓ 2 tbsp olive oil
- ✓ 2 large onions, sliced
- ✓ Sea salt and ground black pepper, to taste
- ✓ 1 thyme sprig, chopped
- ✓ 1 tbsp balsamic vinegar

Directions:

- ❖ In a medium saucepan, bring the vegetable broth to a boil over medium-high heat. Now, add in the cornmeal, whisking continuously to prevent lumps.
- ❖ Reduce the heat to a simmer. Continue to simmer, whisking periodically, for about 18 minutes, until the mixture has thickened. Stir the vegan butter into the cooked polenta. Spoon the cooked polenta into a lightly greased square baking dish. Cover with the plastic wrap and chill for about 2 hours or until firm.
- ❖ Meanwhile, heat the olive oil in a nonstick skillet over a moderately high heat. Cook the onions for about 3 minutes or until just tender and fragrant.
- ❖ Stir in the salt, black pepper, thyme and balsamic vinegar and continue to sauté for 1 minute or so; remove from the heat. Cut your polenta into squares. Spritz a nonstick skillet with a cooking spray. Fry the polenta squares for about 5 minutes per side or until golden brown. Top each polenta toast with the balsamic onion and serve. Enjoy

265)   FREEKEH PILAF WITH CHICKPEAS

Preparation Time: 40 minutes   **Servings: 4**

Ingredients:

- ✓ 4 tbsp olive oil
- ✓ 1 cup shallots, chopped
- ✓ 1 celery stalks, chopped
- ✓ 1 carrot, chopped
- ✓ 1 tsp garlic, minced
- ✓ Sea salt and ground black pepper, to taste
- ✓ 1 tsp cayenne pepper
- ✓ 1 tsp dried basil
- ✓ 1 tsp dried oregano
- ✓ 1 cup freekeh
- ✓ 2 ½ cups water
- ✓ 1 cup boiled chickpeas, drained
- ✓ 2 tbsp roasted peanuts, roughly chopped
- ✓ 2 tbsp fresh mint, roughly chopped

Directions:

- ❖ Heat the olive oil in a heavy-bottomed pot over medium-high heat. Once hot, sauté the shallot, celery and carrot for about 3 minutes until just tender.
- ❖ Then, add in the garlic and continue to sauté for 30 seconds more or until aromatic. Add in the spices, freekeh and water.
- ❖ Turn the heat to a simmer for 30 to 35 minutes, stirring occasionally to promote even cooking. Fold in the boiled chickpeas.
- ❖ To serve, spoon into individual bowls and garnish with roasted peanuts and fresh mint. Enjoy

266)   GRANDMA'S PILAU WITH GARDEN VEGETABLES

Preparation Time: 45 minutes   **Servings: 4**

Ingredients:

- ✓ 2 tbsp olive oil
- ✓ 1 onion, chopped
- ✓ 1 carrot, trimmed and grated
- ✓ 1 parsnip, trimmed and grated
- ✓ 1 celery with leaves, chopped
- ✓ 1 tsp garlic, chopped
- ✓ 1 cup brown rice
- ✓ 2 cups vegetable broth
- ✓ 2 tbsp fresh parsley, chopped
- ✓ 2 tbsp finely basil, chopped

Directions:

- ❖ Heat the olive oil in a saucepan over medium-high heat.
- ❖ Once hot, cook the onion, carrot, parsnip and celery for about 3 minutes until just tender. Add in the garlic and continue to sauté for 1 minute or so until aromatic.
- ❖ In a lightly oiled casserole dish, place the rice, flowed by the sautéed vegetables and broth.
- ❖ Bake, covered, at 375 degrees F for about 40 minutes, stirring after 20 minutes.
- ❖ Garnish with fresh parsley and basil and serve warm. Enjoy

267)   EASY BARLEY RISOTTO

Preparation Time: 35 minutes   **Servings: 4**

Ingredients:

- ✓ 2 tbsp vegan butter
- ✓ 1 medium onion, chopped
- ✓ 1 bell pepper, seeded and chopped
- ✓ 2 garlic cloves, minced
- ✓ 1 tsp ginger, minced
- ✓ 2 cups vegetable broth
- ✓ 2 cups water
- ✓ 1 cup medium pearl barley
- ✓ 1/2 cup white wine
- ✓ 2 tbsp fresh chives, chopped

Directions:

- ❖ Melt the vegan butter in a saucepan over medium-high heat.
- ❖ Once hot, cook the onion and pepper for about 3 minutes until just tender.
- ❖ Add in the garlic and ginger and continue to sauté for 2 minutes or until aromatic.
- ❖ Add in the vegetable broth, water, barley and wine; cover and continue to simmer for about 30 minutes. Once all the liquid has been absorbed; fluff the barley with a fork.
- ❖ Garnish with fresh chives and serve warm. Enjoy

268)   TRADITIONAL PORTUGUESE PAPAS

Preparation Time: 35 minutes   **Servings: 4**

Ingredients:

- ✓ 4 cups water
- ✓ 2 cups rice milk
- ✓ 1 cup grits
- ✓ 1/4 tsp grated nutmeg
- ✓ 1/4 tsp kosher salt
- ✓ 4 tbsp vegan butter
- ✓ 1/4 cup maple syrup

Directions:

- ❖ Bring the water and milk to a boil over a moderately high heat.
- ❖ Stir in the grits, nutmeg and salt. Turn the heat to a simmer, cover and continue to cook, for about 30 minutes or until cooked through.
- ❖ Stir in the vegan butter and maple syrup. Enjoy

269)   THE BEST MILLET PATTIES EVER

Preparation Time: 40 minutes   **Servings: 4**

Ingredients:

- ✓ 1 cup millet
- ✓ 3 cups water
- ✓ 2 tbsp olive oil
- ✓ 1 onion, finely chopped
- ✓ 2 cloves garlic, crushed
- ✓ 1 tsp smoked paprika
- ✓ 1/2 tsp ground cumin
- ✓ Sea salt and ground black pepper, to taste

Directions:

- ❖ Bring the millet and water to a boil; turn the heat to a simmer and continue to cook for 30 minutes.
- ❖ Fluff your millet with a fork and combine it with the remaining ingredients, except for the oil. Shape the mixture into patties.
- ❖ Heat the olive oil in a nonstick skillet over medium-high heat. Fry the patties for 5 minutes per side or until golden-brown and cooked through. Enjoy

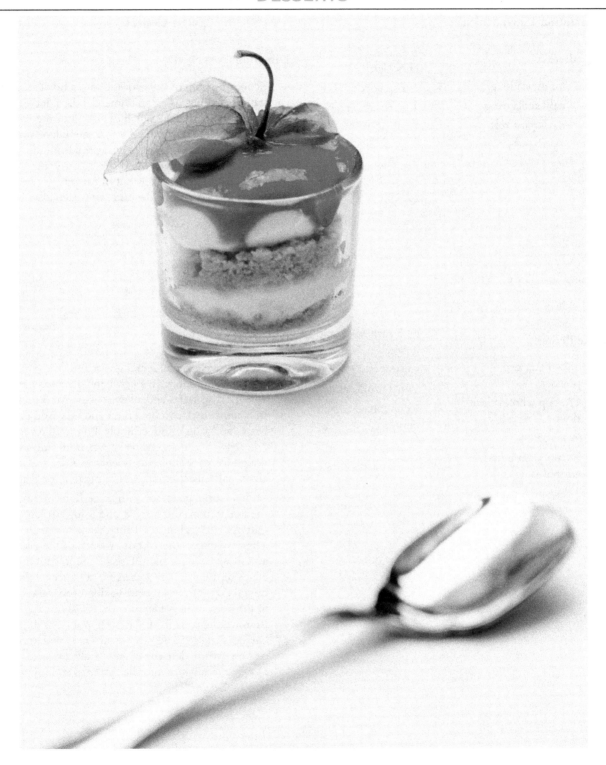

270) AVOCADO TRUFFLES WITH CHOCOLATE COATING

Preparation Time: 5 minutes

Servings: 6

Ingredients:

- ✓ 1 ripe avocado, pitted
- ✓ ½ tsp vanilla extract
- ✓ ½ tsp lemon zest
- ✓ 5 oz dairy-free dark chocolate
- ✓ 1 tbsp coconut oil
- ✓ 1 tbsp unsweetened cocoa powder

Directions:

- ❖ Scoop the pulp of the avocado into a bowl and mix with the vanilla using an immersion blender. Stir in the lemon zest and a pinch of salt. Pour the chocolate and coconut oil into a safe microwave bowl and melt in the microwave for 1 minute. Add to the avocado mixture and stir. Allow cooling to firm up a bit. Form balls out of the mix. Roll each ball in the cocoa powder and serve immediately

271) VANILLA BERRY TARTS

Preparation Time: 35 minutes +

cooling time

Servings: 4

Ingredients:

- ✓ 4 tbsp flaxseed powder
- ✓ 1/3 cup whole-wheat flour
- ✓ ½ tsp salt
- ✓ ¼ cup plant butter, crumbled
- ✓ 3 tbsp pure malt syrup
- ✓ 6 oz cashew cream
- ✓ 6 tbsp pure date sugar
- ✓ ¾ tsp vanilla extract
- ✓ 1 cup mixed frozen berries

Directions:

- ❖ Preheat oven to 350 F and grease mini pie pans with cooking spray. In a bowl, mix flaxseed powder with 12 tbsp water and allow soaking for 5 minutes. In a large bowl, combine flour and salt. Add in butter and whisk until crumbly. Pour in the vegan "flax egg" and malt syrup and mix until smooth dough forms. Flatten the dough on a flat surface, cover with plastic wrap, and refrigerate for 1 hour.
- ❖ Dust a working surface with some flour, remove the dough onto the surface, and using a rolling pin, flatten the dough into a 1-inch diameter circle. Use a large cookie cutter, cut out rounds of the dough and fit into the pie pans. Use a knife to trim the edges of the pan. Lay a parchment paper on the dough cups, pour on some baking beans, and bake in the oven until golden brown, 15-20 minutes. Remove the pans from the oven, pour out the baking beans, and allow cooling. In a bowl, mix cashew cream, date sugar, and vanilla extract. Divide the mixture into the tart cups and top with berries. Serve

272) HOMEMADE CHOCOLATES WITH COCONUT AND RAISINS

Preparation Time: 10 minutes +

chilling time

Servings: 20

Ingredients:

- ✓ 1/2 cup cacao butter, melted
- ✓ 1/3 cup peanut butter
- ✓ 1/4 cup agave syrup
- ✓ A pinch of grated nutmeg
- ✓ A pinch of coarse salt
- ✓ 1/2 tsp vanilla extract
- ✓ 1 cup dried coconut, shredded
- ✓ 6 ounces dark chocolate, chopped
- ✓ 3 ounces raisins

Directions:

- ❖ Thoroughly combine all the ingredients, except for the chocolate, in a mixing bowl.
- ❖ Spoon the mixture into molds. Leave to set hard in a cool place.
- ❖ Melt the dark chocolate in your microwave. Pour in the melted chocolate until the fillings are covered. Leave to set hard in a cool place.
- ❖ Enjoy

273) MOCHA FUDGE

Preparation Time: 1 hour 10

minutes

Servings: 20

Ingredients:

- ✓ 1 cup cookies, crushed
- ✓ 1/2 cup almond butter
- ✓ 1/4 cup agave nectar
- ✓ 6 ounces dark chocolate, broken into chunks
- ✓ 1 tsp instant coffee
- ✓ A pinch of grated nutmeg
- ✓ A pinch of salt

Directions:

- ❖ Line a large baking sheet with parchment paper.
- ❖ Melt the chocolate in your microwave and add in the remaining ingredients; stir to combine well.
- ❖ Scrape the batter into a parchment-lined baking sheet. Place it in your freezer for at least 1 hour to set.
- ❖ Cut into squares and serve. Enjoy

274) ALMOND AND CHOCOLATE CHIP BARS

Preparation Time: 40 minutes

Servings: 10

Ingredients:

- ✓ 1/2 cup almond butter
- ✓ 1/4 cup coconut oil, melted
- ✓ 1/4 cup agave syrup
- ✓ 1 tsp vanilla extract
- ✓ 1/4 tsp sea salt
- ✓ 1/4 tsp grated nutmeg
- ✓ 1/2 tsp ground cinnamon
- ✓ 2 cups almond flour
- ✓ 1/4 cup flaxseed meal
- ✓ 1 cup vegan chocolate, cut into chunks
- ✓ 1 1/3 cups almonds, ground
- ✓ 2 tbsp cacao powder
- ✓ 1/4 cup agave syrup

Directions:

- ❖ In a mixing bowl, thoroughly combine the almond butter, coconut oil, 1/4 cup of agave syrup, vanilla, salt, nutmeg and cinnamon.
- ❖ Gradually stir in the almond flour and flaxseed meal and stir to combine. Add in the chocolate chunks and stir again.
- ❖ In a small mixing bowl, combine the almonds, cacao powder and agave syrup. Now, spread the ganache onto the cake. Freeze for about 30 minutes, cut into bars and serve well chilled. Enjoy

275)   ALMOND BUTTER COOKIES

Preparation Time: 45 minutes

Servings: 10

Ingredients:

- ✓ 3/4 cup all-purpose flour
- ✓ 1/2 tsp baking soda
- ✓ 1/4 tsp kosher salt
- ✓ 1 flax egg
- ✓ 1/4 cup coconut oil, at room temperature
- ✓ 2 tbsp almond milk
- ✓ 1/2 cup brown sugar
- ✓ 1/2 cup almond butter
- ✓ 1/2 tsp ground cinnamon
- ✓ 1/2 tsp vanilla

Directions:

- ❖ In a mixing bowl, combine the flour, baking soda and salt.
- ❖ In another bowl, combine the flax egg, coconut oil, almond milk, sugar, almond butter, cinnamon and vanilla. Stir the wet mixture into the dry ingredients and stir until well combined.
- ❖ Place the batter in your refrigerator for about 30 minutes. Shape the batter into small cookies and arrange them on a parchment-lined cookie pan.
- ❖ Bake in the preheated oven at 350 degrees F for approximately 12 minutes. Transfer the pan to a wire rack to cool at room temperature. Enjoy

276)   PEANUT BUTTER OATMEAL BARS

Preparation Time: 25 minutes

Servings: 20

Ingredients:

- ✓ 1 cup vegan butter
- ✓ 3/4 cup coconut sugar
- ✓ 2 tbsp applesauce
- ✓ 1 ¾ cups old-fashioned oats
- ✓ 1 tsp baking soda
- ✓ A pinch of sea salt
- ✓ A pinch of grated nutmeg
- ✓ 1 tsp pure vanilla extract
- ✓ 1 cup oat flour
- ✓ 1 cup all-purpose flour

Directions:

- ❖ Begin by preheating your oven to 350 degrees F.
- ❖ In a mixing bowl, thoroughly combine the dry ingredients. In another bowl, combine the wet ingredients.
- ❖ Then, stir the wet mixture into the dry ingredients; mix to combine well.
- ❖ Spread the batter mixture in a parchment-lined square baking pan. Bake in the preheated oven for about 20 minutes. Enjoy

277)   VANILLA HALVAH FUDGE

Preparation Time: 10 minutes +

chilling time

Servings: 16

Ingredients:

- ✓ 1/2 cup cocoa butter
- ✓ 1/2 cup tahini
- ✓ 8 dates, pitted
- ✓ 1/4 tsp ground cloves
- ✓ A pinch of grated nutmeg
- ✓ A pinch coarse salt
- ✓ 1 tsp vanilla extract

Directions:

- ❖ Line a square baking pan with parchment paper.
- ❖ Mix the ingredients until everything is well incorporated.
- ❖ Scrape the batter into the parchment-lined pan. Place in your freezer until ready to serve. Enjoy

278)   RAW CHOCOLATE MANGO PIE

Preparation Time: 10 minutes +

chilling time

Servings: 16

Ingredients:

- ✓ Avocado layer:
- ✓ 3 ripe avocados, pitted and peeled
- ✓ A pinch of sea salt
- ✓ A pinch of ground anise
- ✓ 1/2 tsp vanilla paste
- ✓ 2 tbsp coconut milk
- ✓ 5 tbsp agave syrup
- ✓ 1/3 cup cocoa powder
- ✓ Crema layer:
- ✓ 1/3 cup almond butter
- ✓ 1/2 cup coconut cream
- ✓ 1 medium mango, peeled
- ✓ 1/2 coconut flakes
- ✓ 2 tbsp agave syrup

Directions:

- ❖ In your food processor, blend the avocado layer until smooth and uniform, reserve.
- ❖ Then, blend the other layer in a separate bowl. Spoon the layers in a lightly oiled baking pan.
- ❖ Transfer the cake to your freezer for about 3 hours. Store in your freezer. Enjoy

279)   CHOCOLATE N'ICE CREAM

Preparation Time: 10 minutes

Servings: 1

Ingredients:

- ✓ 2 frozen bananas, peeled and sliced
- ✓ 2 tbsp coconut milk
- ✓ 1 tsp carob powder
- ✓ 1 tsp cocoa powder
- ✓ A pinch of grated nutmeg
- ✓ 1/8 tsp ground cardamom
- ✓ 1/8 tsp ground cinnamon
- ✓ 1 tbsp chocolate curls

Directions:

- ❖ Place all the ingredients in the bowl of your food processor or high-speed blender.
- ❖ Blitz the ingredients until creamy or until your desired consistency is achieved.
- ❖ Serve immediately or store in your freezer.
- ❖ Enjoy

280)   RAW RASPBERRY CHEESECAKE

Preparation Time: 15 minutes +

chilling time

Servings: 9

Ingredients:

- ✓ Crust:
- ✓ 2 cups almonds
- ✓ 1 cup fresh dates, pitted
- ✓ 1/4 tsp ground cinnamon

- ✓ Filling:
- ✓ 2 cups raw cashews, soaked overnight and drained
- ✓ 14 ounces blackberries, frozen
- ✓ 1 tbsp fresh lime juice
- ✓ 1/4 tsp crystallized ginger
- ✓ 1 can coconut cream
- ✓ 8 fresh dates, pitted

Directions:

- ❖ In your food processor, blend the crust ingredients until the mixture comes together; press the crust into a lightly oiled springform pan.
- ❖ Then, blend the filling layer until completely smooth. Spoon the filling onto the crust, creating a flat surface with a spatula.
- ❖ Transfer the cake to your freezer for about 3 hours. Store in your freezer.
- ❖ Garnish with organic citrus peel. Enjoy

281)   MINI LEMON TARTS

Preparation Time: 15 minutes +

chilling time

Servings: 9

Ingredients:

- ✓ 1 cup cashews
- ✓ 1 cup dates, pitted
- ✓ 1/2 cup coconut flakes

- ✓ 1/2 tsp anise, ground
- ✓ 3 lemons, freshly squeezed
- ✓ 1 cup coconut cream
- ✓ 2 tbsp agave syrup

Directions:

- ❖ Brush a muffin tin with a nonstick cooking oil.
- ❖ Blend the cashews, dates, coconut and anise in your food processor or a high-speed blender. Press the crust into the peppered muffin tin.
- ❖ Then, blend the lemon, coconut cream and agave syrup. Spoon the cream into the muffin tin.
- ❖ Store in your freezer. Enjoy

282) COCONUT BLONDIES WITH RAISINS

Preparation Time: 30 minutes

Servings: 9

Ingredients:

- ✓ 1 cup coconut flour
- ✓ 1 cup all-purpose flour
- ✓ 1/2 tsp baking powder
- ✓ 1/4 tsp salt
- ✓ 1 cup desiccated coconut, unsweetened
- ✓ 3/4 cup vegan butter, softened
- ✓ 1 ½ cups brown sugar
- ✓ 3 tbsp applesauce
- ✓ 1/2 tsp vanilla extract
- ✓ 1/2 tsp ground anise
- ✓ 1 cup raisins, soaked for 15 minutes

Directions:

- ❖ Start by preheating your oven to 350 degrees F. Brush a baking pan with a nonstick cooking oil.
- ❖ Thoroughly combine the flour, baking powder, salt and coconut. In another bowl, mix the butter, sugar, applesauce, vanilla and anise. Stir the butter mixture into the dry ingredients; stir to combine well.
- ❖ Fold in the raisins. Press the batter into the prepared baking pan.
- ❖ Bake for approximately 25 minutes or until it is set in the middle. Place the cake on a wire rack to cool slightly.
- ❖ Enjoy

283) CHOCOLATE SQUARES

Preparation Time: 1 hour 10 minutes

Servings: 20

Ingredients:

- ✓ 1 cup cashew butter
- ✓ 1 cup almond butter
- ✓ 1/4 cup coconut oil, melted
- ✓ 1/4 cup raw cacao powder
- ✓ 2 ounces dark chocolate
- ✓ 4 tbsp agave syrup
- ✓ 1 tsp vanilla paste
- ✓ 1/4 tsp ground cinnamon
- ✓ 1/4 tsp ground cloves

Directions:

- ❖ Process all the ingredients in your blender until uniform and smooth.
- ❖ Scrape the batter into a parchment-lined baking sheet. Place it in your freezer for at least 1 hour to set.
- ❖ Cut into squares and serve. Enjoy

284) CHOCOLATE AND RAISIN COOKIE BARS

Preparation Time: 40 minutes

Servings: 10

Ingredients:

- ✓ 1/2 cup peanut butter, at room temperature
- ✓ 1 cup agave syrup
- ✓ 1 tsp pure vanilla extract
- ✓ 1/4 tsp kosher salt
- ✓ 2 cups almond flour
- ✓ 1 tsp baking soda
- ✓ 1 cup raisins
- ✓ 1 cup vegan chocolate, broken into chunks

Directions:

- ❖ In a mixing bowl, thoroughly combine the peanut butter, agave syrup, vanilla and salt.
- ❖ Gradually stir in the almond flour and baking soda and stir to combine. Add in the raisins and chocolate chunks and stir again.
- ❖ Freeze for about 30 minutes and serve well chilled. Enjoy

285) ALMOND GRANOLA BARS

Preparation Time: 25 minutes

Servings: 12

Ingredients:

- ✓ 1/2 cup spelt flour
- ✓ 1/2 cup oat flour
- ✓ 1 cup rolled oats
- ✓ 1 tsp baking powder
- ✓ 1/2 tsp cinnamon
- ✓ 1/2 tsp ground cardamom
- ✓ 1/4 tsp freshly grated nutmeg
- ✓ 1/8 tsp kosher salt
- ✓ 1 cup almond milk
- ✓ 3 tbsp agave syrup
- ✓ 1/2 cup peanut butter
- ✓ 1/2 cup applesauce
- ✓ 1/2 tsp pure almond extract
- ✓ 1/2 tsp pure vanilla extract
- ✓ 1/2 cup almonds, slivered

Directions:

- ❖ Begin by preheating your oven to 350 degrees F.
- ❖ In a mixing bowl, thoroughly combine the flour, oats, baking powder and spices. In another bowl, combine the wet ingredients.
- ❖ Then, stir the wet mixture into the dry ingredients; mix to combine well. Fold in the slivered almonds.
- ❖ Scrape the batter mixture into a parchment-lined baking pan. Bake in the preheated oven for about 20 minutes. Let it cool on a wire rack. Cut into bars and enjoy

286)   COCONUT COOKIES

Preparation Time: 40 minutes

Servings: 10

Ingredients:

- ✓ 1/2 cup oat flour
- ✓ 1/2 cup all-purpose flour
- ✓ 1/2 tsp baking soda
- ✓ A pinch of salt
- ✓ 1/4 tsp grated nutmeg
- ✓ 1/2 tsp ground cloves
- ✓ 1/2 tsp ground cinnamon
- ✓ 4 tbsp coconut oil
- ✓ 2 tbsp oat milk
- ✓ 1/2 cup coconut sugar
- ✓ 1/2 cup coconut flakes, unsweetened

Directions:

- ❖ In a mixing bowl, combine the flour, baking soda and spices.
- ❖ In another bowl, combine the coconut oil, oat milk, sugar and coconut. Stir the wet mixture into the dry ingredients and stir until well combined.
- ❖ Place the batter in your refrigerator for about 30 minutes. Shape the batter into small cookies and arrange them on a parchment-lined cookie pan.
- ❖ Bake in the preheated oven at 330 degrees F for approximately 10 minutes. Transfer the pan to a wire rack to cool at room temperature. Enjoy

287)   RAW WALNUT AND BERRY CAKE

Preparation Time: 10 minutes +

chilling time

Servings: 8

Ingredients:

- ✓ Crust:
- ✓ 1 ½ cups walnuts, ground
- ✓ 2 tbsp maple syrup
- ✓ 1/4 cup raw cacao powder
- ✓ 1/4 tsp ground cinnamon
- ✓ A pinch of coarse salt
- ✓ A pinch of freshly grated nutmeg
- ✓ Berry layer:
- ✓ 6 cups mixed berries
- ✓ 2 frozen bananas
- ✓ 1/2 cup agave syrup

Directions:

- ❖ In your food processor, blend the crust ingredients until the mixture comes together; press the crust into a lightly oiled baking pan.
- ❖ Then, blend the berry layer. Spoon the berry layer onto the crust, creating a flat surface with a spatula.
- ❖ Transfer the cake to your freezer for about 3 hours. Store in your freezer. Enjoy

AUTHOR BIOGRAPHY

THE PLANT-BASED DIET COOKBOOK

Cook Your Green Passion: 100+ New Tasty Recipes to Try on All Occasions!

THE PLANT-BASED DIET

Cookbook for Beginners

THE PLANT-BASED DIET FOR WOMEN

Simple, Healthy Recipes to Rise Your Everyday Energy and Balance Hormones!

THE PLANT-BASED DIET COOKBOOK FOR ATHLETE

Guide and 100+ Tasty Recipes for a Strong Body and a Healthy Life. Lose Weight and Shape the Body, for Beginners and Experts of All Sports.

THE PLANT-BASED DIET RECIPE BOOK:

2 Books in 1: Easy Beginner's Cookbook with Plant-Based Recipes for Healthy Eating

THE PLANT-BASED DIET FOR BEGINNERS' WOMEN:

2 Books in 1: A Special Guide for Beginners with More than 200 Simple, Healthy Recipes to Rise Your Everyday Energy and Balance Hormones!

THE PLANT-BASED FOR ATHLETE:

2 Books in 1: All You Need to Know About the Plant-Based Diet + More Than 200 Tasty Recipes for a Strong Body and a Healthy Life. Lose Weight and Shape the Body, for Beginners and Experts of All Sports!

THE PLANT-BASED DIET QUICK & EASY:

2 Books in 1: 220+ New Delicious Vegan and Vegetarian Quick & Easy-to-Follow Recipe to Taste!

THE PLANT-BASED DIET FOR MEN:

2 Books in 1: A Game-Changing Approach to Peak Performance! Guide for Beginners: 240+ Quick & Easy, Affordable Recipes that Novice and Busy People Can Do! Reset and Energize Your Body!

THE PLANT-BASED DIET FOR FITNESS:

2 Books in 1: The revolutionary diet book with easy and tasty recipes for healthy and smart people! 240 Fantastic Recipes to Get Fit and Lose Weight!

THE MASTER PLANT-BASED DIET:

3 Books in 1: The Master Guide for Beginners for Vegetarians & Vegans! Try and Taste More than 350 New Recipes and Get to Know About How this Diet Can Help You as Men or Women and Athlete! Special Chapters inside!!!

THE PLANT-BASED DIET FOR BODYBUILDING:

3 Books in 1: 350 Recipes All Vegan & Vegetarian with High-Protein! Beginners Guide to Increase Muscle Mass with Healthy and Whole-Food Vegan Recipes to Fuel Your Workouts!

THE COMPLETE DIET FOR ABSOLUTE BEGINNERS ON PLANT-BASED DIET:

4 Books in 1: Cookbook for Beginners: 470+ Meals to Energize Your Body and Fuel Your Workouts with High-Protein Vegan and Vegetarian Recipes, Healthy and Whole Foods Recipes to Kick-Start a Healthy Eating!

THE PLANT-BASED DIET FOR ONE:

The Revolutionary Recipe Book with Easy and Tasty Recipes for Healthy Lifestyle and Smart People! Lose Rapidly Weight with a Large Choice of 120+ Vegan and Vegetarian Recipes!

THE PLANT-BASED DIET LIKE A RESTAURANT

2 Books in 1: Cook Vegetarian and Vegan Choosing Among Special and Delicious Recipes Like a Chef! Live a Healthy Lifestyle and Lose Rapidly Weight with a Large Choice of 240+ Vegan and Vegetarian Recipes!

THE PLANT-BASED DIET BASICS:

2 Books in 1: All You Need to Know About the Plant-Based Diet + More Than 240 Delicious Vegan and Vegetarian Recipes for Weight Loss and Live Healthy!

THE PLANT-BASED DIET FOR SINGLE:

2 Books in 1: Live a Healthy Lifestyle and Lose Rapidly Weight with a Large Choice of 240+ Vegan and Vegetarian Recipes! Special Guide Included!

THE PLANT-BASED DIET FOR WEIGHT LOSS:

2 Books in 1: Cookbook for Beginners: 240+ Vegetarian and Vegan Recipes to Energize Your Body and Get to Know About How this Diet Can Help to Lose Weight!

THE PLANT-BASED DIET FOR WOMEN OVER 50

3 Books in 1: The Guide and Cookbook for a Simple and Healthy 340+ Recipes to Rise Your Everyday Energy and Balance Hormones!

THE PLANT-BASED DIET FOR MEN OVER 50:

3 Books in 1: A Game-Changing Approach to Peak Performance! 340+ New Delicious Vegan and Vegetarian Quick & Easy-to-Follow Recipe!

THE MASTER EDITION OF PLANT-BASED DIET:

4 Books in 1: A Game-Changing Approach to Peak Performance! 450+ Recipes All Vegan & Vegetarian with High-Protein! Beginners Guide to Live a Healthy Lifestyle! Whole-Food Vegan and Vegetarian Recipes!

CPSIA information can be obtained
at www.ICGtesting.com
Printed in the USA
BVHW051258250521
608095BV00006B/1838